Raquel Lopes Rios

The construction of identity in relation to the other

Raquel Lopes Rios

The construction of identity in relation to the other

A discussion based on a reading of the short stories in Clarice Lispector's "Beauty and the Beast"

ScienciaScripts

Imprint

Cover image: Provided by the author

This book is a translation from the original published under ISBN 978-613-9-68524-0.

Publisher:
Sciencia Scripts
is a trademark of
Dodo Books Indian Ocean Ltd. and OmniScriptum S.R.L publishing group

120 High Road, East Finchley, London, N2 9ED, United Kingdom
Str. Armeneasca 28/1, office 1, Chisinau MD-2012, Republic of Moldova, Europe
Printed at: see last page
ISBN: 978-620-7-72892-3

To my family, the greatest example of hard work and dedication, a safe haven with unconditional love, a source of inspiration.

ACKNOWLEDGMENTS

First of all to God, whose presence I have felt and feel in every step of this arduous journey, as well as in every second of my life.

To my parents, who believe in and give wings to my dreams, sparing no effort to make each one of them come true.

To my brothers, my sister-in-law, my niece and the rest of my family, who, even though they are far away, are present with immeasurable affection and generosity.

To Marcia Marques, who with wisdom and affection accompanied and guided me throughout this process.

To Ivete Lara Camargos Walty, who was responsible for presenting the short story *Beauty and the Beast or The Wound Too Big,* in one of her postgraduate classes.

To Arthur Parreiras Gomes, who, while still an undergraduate in psychology, awakened me to the possibility of going down new paths and sparked my interest in literature even more.

To Gisele Britto, the true meeting of the analytical pair, who makes it possible for me every day to have greater contact with the other and, above all, with myself.

To my patients, my daily source of learning and passion.

To my friends, for their companionship and delicious moments of relaxation and reflection.

To my colleagues in the master's courses and to the professors for their welcome, teachings and exchanges.

CAPES for the encouragement and financial support of the scholarship.

To the Letters Postgraduate Program and to everyone who made this stage possible.

How can I understand myself? Why that blind integration at first? And then the near-joy of liberation? What material am I made of, where the elements and the basis of a thousand other lives are intertwined but not fused? I follow all the paths and none of them is mine yet. I've been molded into so many statues and I've never stood still [...] (LISPECTOR, 1979, p. 77).

SUMMARY

This paper seeks to broaden the discussion about the formation of identity in the relationship with the other, based on a reading of the short stories in Clarice Lispector's *Beauty and the Beast*. The choice of this work as the object of study is mainly due to the fact that in these short stories the characters' search for recognition of themselves and their own identity recurs. In addition, we believe that not only does the text contain elements that support our discussion, but also the processes of writing and reading it. In analyzing the short stories, we adopted psychoanalytic theory, which, like literature, affirms the power of the unconscious in human motivations and endorses the importance of affections, fantasies and desires in the process of subjectivation. Faced with the variety of possible meanings for the concept of identity, for this work we will adopt its definition from a psychoanalytic point of view, following the changes in the conception of the subject that Freudian discoveries have brought about. All this with the aim of opening up new interpretative paths for the literary text and, consequently, creating new conditions for us to think about other ways of enunciating the self and positioning ourselves in relation to the world and the other. We realized that, although the literary text is a space that allows for many interpretations, it is still incapable of transmitting all that reality entails and, in this way, recognizes the limits of representation and language, making this a cause for creation. Similarly, it is from his own lack and emptiness that the subject will move towards the creation of his own identity, and this is one of the points of greatest convergence with literary art.

Keywords: Literature. Psychoanalysis. Identity. Clarice Lispector. Otherness.

SUMMARY

INTRODUCED

From that moment when we too take a risk, it is no longer a fact to tell, there is a lack of words that would not betray it. (LISPECTOR,1964,p.99)

The constant human search to establish meanings and definitions implies a permanent question in contemporary times: what is identity? Inserted in a context of increasing globalization, it is also necessary to demarcate territories and traces of singularity.

Despite the great scientific and technological advances in countless areas of knowledge, we still ask ourselves, as сото о we have done for centuries: who are we; what kind of bond binds us to the other, be it family, neighbor or stranger?

O *Diciondrio Aurelio* (2010) gives us just two meanings for identity, which is enough to immerse us in the ambiguity and complexity that surrounds this concept of identity, namely: "1. quality of being identical; 2. proper and exclusive characteristics of a person: поте, age, status, profession." (p. 406). So we ask ourselves: Is it possible for a characteristic to be exclusive and, at the same time, identical to something else? Is it possible to establish a stable meaning for the very notion of identity?

Joel Birman and Eduardo Leal Cunha, both psychoanalysts and scholars of "identity", state that this is an underdeveloped and poorly understood concept, and that, currently, the discussion about it is almost always based on the perspective of its de-centering, which is linked to the de-centering or displacement of another notion that is central to modem thought: the idea of the subject.

Birman (2003b), in his book *Freud and Philosophy,* proposes a discussion about the transformations brought about by psychoanalysis, one of which is the deconstruction of the category of subject through its decentering. According to him, at the end of the 19th century, the great influence of Freudian thought contributed to a deconstruction of the Cartesian *cogito,* causing concrete impacts on subjectivities and, therefore, on what can be thought of as identity, creating the conditions for us to think of other ways of enunciating the self and positioning ourselves in relation to the world and the other. For Birman (2003), this decentering took place in three movements: from consciousness to the unconscious; from the self to the other; and from representation to drive.

In the first chapter of this work, we will discuss the first Freudian decentering, in which consciousness was removed from its prominent place in the psyche and relativized in relation to the unconscious. The discovery of the unconscious made possible new productions of meaning, new modes of subjectivation, in which fantasy and affect produce effects beyond rational thought. These effects can be identified in Clarice's characters, and also in the reader, by reading the stories in *Beauty and the Beast, the* subject of our study. Among these effects, the strangeness caused by the encounter with something familiar, which ambiguously turns into its opposite, is highlighted in this chapter. We believe that the strangeness of reading the text, as well as the restlessness of some of the characters described in the narratives, are indicators of hidden elements that need to be awakened in order to discuss our theme.

The method of interpretation proposed by Freud, based on the discovery of the unconscious, then implies the construction of meaning in the relationship with the Other, leading us to think of the second movement of decentering: from the self to the other. Freudian discourse formulated that "the self, as the totalizing instantiation of the psyche and the body, would not be original, as previously thought, but derived from the investment of the other" (BIRMAN, 2003, p. 66). With this new shift in the category of subject brought about by Freudian thought, the forms of relationship with otherness are also transformed, so that the recognition of self and other becomes interdependent. This intimate encounter between the self and the other is initially described in the second chapter from a psychoanalytical point of view and then transcends this description when we identify it in the literary text. The analysis of the short stories makes it possible to understand how the characters are constituted through their relationship with other characters, how the narrator constructs his narrative and also how the reader is constituted in this intersubjective relationship with the text. Furthermore, we believe that the literature figure сото an other for psychoanalysis, serving сото model, auxiliary and even rival to Freudian thought, thus participating in the birth of psychoanalytic theory itself.

In the third chapter of this work, we will see the impossibility of representation being able to integrate the subject's experience in the relationship with himself and with the other; it will then be with the introduction of the notion of the death drive, a drive without representation, pure force in movement and producer of rupture and dispersion, that Freudian thought will operate the third movement: from representation to drive. For Birman (2003):

> This de-centering called into question the attribute of representation, which in turn was no longer intrinsic to the order of life. This would now be crossed by death, the insistent power of discord, always disarticulating the order of life and requiring it to permanently reconstruct itself in the face of the transgressions promoted by discord. If rcprcscntation is a production of Eros, the death drive would always aim to deconstruct the established rcprcscntacocs, demanding new connections and the production of other psychic rcprcscntacocs (p. 70).

Thus, a permanent war between love and discord insists on being instituted in the psyche, "so that representing how this war takes place is no longer an easy possibility for subjectivity." (BIRMAN, 2003, p. 71). It's no longer an easy possibility, nor is it impossible, especially when we're dealing with new forms of relationship with otherness, including the relationship between different types of knowledge and, to this end, we call on the rich contribution of art, especially literature.

When we talk about the drive and the resulting combinatorial games of representations, we are consequently referring to the production of fantasies, since "the work of fantasizing is, therefore, precisely the permanent ordering and reordering of these movements and limits in a network of representations: constructing at every moment the meeting point between the demands of the drive and the limits imposed by the other." (CUNHA, 2005, p. 191). It's in this way that fantasies unfold in narrative forms that try to account, in a unique way, for each person's apprehension of reality.

In this way, literature and psychoanalysis come together in that they are not bound by the positivist knowledge of science and seek to explore the unpredictable and unsustainable nature of human experience and desire. As Teixeira (2005) states:

> The literary experience of language is expressed through the tragicity and transgression that it carries within itself, subverting, contesting, threatening the author, reader and even the work: it is a place of apprehension of meaning, of epiphanies, of the inapprehensible, of desire, in which poetic invention is the most representative example (p. 5).

Literature and psychoanalysis appear to be mutually supportive in affirming the power of the unconscious in human motivations and, consequently, that life is an enigma. We followed the intensity of the power of literature, which Freud affirmed as a source of knowledge, and then chose the literary work *Beauty and the Beast* by Clarice Lispector as the object of study for this paper.

Even though Clarice herself declared: "Don't worry about understanding. Living surpasses any understanding" (LISPECTOR, 1998a, back cover), her words do make it possible to "understand" ourselves...

In this work, we will seek, in particular, to understand more about the construction of identity in the relationship with the other, paying attention to the author's "form" of writing, a fundamental aspect in achieving this objective.

A bela e a fera, published in 1979 by Nova Fronteira, is an organization of Clarice Lispector's short stories by Olga Borelli, a friend, collaborator and companion during the last years of the writer's life. The posthumous book brings together eight unpublished short stories, entitled *Historia interrompida, Gertrudespede um conselho, Obsessao, O delirio, A fuga, Mais dois bebados, Um dia a menos and A bela e a fera ou a ferida grande demais.* The first six stories are included in the first part of the book, as they were written by Clarice as a teenager in the 1940s, and the other two were the last stories written by the author in 1977, the year of her death.

The fact that the work groups together short stories written at different times in the author's life also allows us to think about a process of representation of the identity of Clarice's own writing, paying attention to changes and similarities in the writing throughout the work.

Finally, recognizing the limits of representation and, consequently, of language, as well as our limits in studying the subject, doesn't stop us from thinking even more about it and producing something around this permanent question: who am I?

Warned that, at the end of the work, we probably won't get a single answer to this ongoing question, we are left with the proposal to follow the paths that led us to this question, driven by Clarice Lispector's literature.

1 FROM THE CONSCIOUS TO THE UNCONSCIOUS

> *Above all, they had awakened in me the sensation that a deeper and more intense life was beating in my body and spirit than the one I was living (LISPECTOR, 1979, p. 69).*

1.1 The Freudian discovery

Reading and analyzing the short stories in *The Beauty and the Beast* by Clarisse Lispector aroused our concern not only because of the content of the text, which allows us to reflect on the theme of the construction of identity, but also because of the process of reading and writing itself, which covers important aspects for discussing this theme. Of course, as one of the different ways of enunciating the self, literary writing has not been immune to transformations in the notion of subject and identity; on the contrary, it has staged and is staging these aspects in a way that transcends the limits of science and language itself.

Faced with the multiplicity of paths to be taken, and the multiplicity of possible readings and interpretations of a literary text, we will adopt the psychoanalytic approach to our reading, so as not to get lost in this labyrinth of possibilities. This is because we believe that the dialogue between psychoanalysis and literature will take us through privileged paths of fantasy production, the journey of desire, encounters with otherness, among other aspects based on the experience of freedom rather than control and predictability. These are aspects that are so dear to the process of subjectivation and which we will be able to understand better throughout this work.

So let's start by clarifying the direction of the movements of de-centering of the idea of the subject operated by psychoanalysis, pointed out by Birman (2003), and then see how the representations contained in literary art transcend such theorizing and broaden the discussion of our theme.

The first movement, according to Birman (2003), was from the conscious to the unconscious. This is because, according to the psychoanalyst, before the Freudian discovery of the unconscious, there was a predominance of thought which he calls "modern rationality", initially marked by absolute belief in the powers of reason and consciousness. This thinking strongly influenced the scientific production of psychiatry and psychology, which identified the psychic with the being of consciousness, and only this was its truth.

The founders of psychiatry, Esquirol and Pinel, stated that mental alienation was due to excessive passions and, as such, pointed to the intemacy of the alienated and to moral treatment as a possible solution, unlike the psychiatry of the Ancien Régime, which said that the loss of reason was unavoidable. Subsequently, biological hypotheses in the form of theories of heredity and degeneration also gained ground, and in all these theories, psychism was restricted to the field of consciousness, so that it would always be the primordial alterations in the brain.

This was not very different in the field of classical psychology, which focused its studies on mental faculties, such as sensation, perception, attention, memory, among others, all of which also refer to consciousness. Furthermore, due to its roots in Descartes' philosophy, the Cartesian *cogito* "I think, therefore I am" defined the category of existence as essentially linked to the register of thought, with imagination often considered a deviation from the straight path of knowledge. This gave daydreams, delusions, hallucinations and other psychic formations a negative and undesirable aspect. In the words of Birman (2003):

> In other words, classical psychiatry and psychology, by restricting themselves to the registers of consciousness, the self and thought in order to conceive of subjectivity, were reduced to the true-false opposition in order to read the disorders of the spirit. There would therefore be no positivity in the experience of madness, but only pure negativity, i.e. in hallucinations and delirium, subjectivity said nothing (p. 23).

However, the Freudian gesture of formulating another psychic register, called the unconscious, "shifted the problem of madness from the register of adequacy, between the self and the object, to that of the production of meaning" (BIRMAN, 2003, p. 25). The discovery of the unconscious and the consequent production of meaning thus expands the forms and possibilities of understanding the human being and their subjectivity.

This brings us closer to our object of study: the literary text. This is because we believe that literature is a vast space for the production of meanings, and we highlight Clarice's writing, recognized by many for its authentic construction of the symbolic universe. Critics consider the fact that, in order to describe the characters and their recurring search for the meaning of life, Clarice makes symbolic use of reality more as a support for the act of searching for fictional subjects than as a historical or geographical reference. Regarding this symbolic use in *Lagos de familia* (LISPECTOR, 1994) and *A legiao estrangeira* (LISPECTOR, 1964), we draw on the considerations of Affonso Romano de Sant'Anna:

> [...] its symbolic universe is only accidentally focused on "reality" as it is codified and defined by the community. His text is not interested in external referents. Geography and history are referred to only accidentally. His literature is not **realistic,** but **symbolic, in that** the text establishes its own referents and is not interested in reflecting the outside world in a mimetic work. (SANT'ANNA, 1990, p. 160, emphasis in original).

Affonso Romano de Sant'Anna's considerations then reiterate our assertion about the possible approximation between literature and psychoanalysis, while at the same time citing aspects of Clarice's writing that justify our choice of one of her works for this paper.

With regard to the rapprochement between literature and psychoanalysis, other relationships are possible; among them, we highlight the work with unconscious aspects. SAMPAIO (2002) states that: "The two fields - that which is constituted between analyst and analysand and that which is engendered between author, text and reader - come closer because they imply an incessant work with language, both allowing themselves to be infiltrated by the unconscious." (p. 159). This statement is endorsed by the writer herself, Clarice Lispector, when she says that: "Sometimes I have the impression that I write out of simple intense curiosity. And that, in writing, I give myself the most unexpected surprises. It's when I write that I often become aware of things that, being unconscious, I didn't know I knew before." (LISPECTOR, 1999a, p. 254).

Furthermore, throughout the work, we will see that the role of the unconscious is not restricted to the act of writing, but involves the act of reading and, consequently, the unconscious issues of the reader as well.

Reiterating the concept of the unconscious in psychoanalysis, let's go back to Birman (2003), when he recalls that Sigmund Freud, through his clinical experience with hysteria - enigmatic precisely because it questioned medicine on its anatomo-clinical basis, together with the method of hypnosis (which taught him the power of language in the production and cure of symptoms) -, he formulated the concept of the unconscious, which was considered to be another field for the production of meaning, bringing to center stage the desires and affections that are fundamental to subjective experience, leading to unique modes of subjectivation.

Eduardo Leal Cunha (2005), another scholar of the perspective of the decentering of the subject and its influence on the constitution of identity, summarizes the effects of Freud's discovery by saying that:

> From the discovery of the unconscious, of another field of meaning production beyond the reach of consciousness and the self, capable, however, of producing effects on the body, and the consequent Freudian formulations about a psychic reality in which fantasy and affections produce concrete effects on subjectivity, The "I" and consciousness lose their prevalent value for animal life and, on the other hand, for sexuality, desires and affections take center stage and fantasy becomes a potency founded on the power of language and the intensities circulating in the psyche. The truth about the subject does not find correspondence or the possibility of verification in so-called material reality, accessible to the self and consciousness, but emerges, often unexpectedly or enigmatically, coro in symptoms and failed acts, in a tangle of fantasies composed of psychic traces impregnated with intensity and force. (CUNHA, 2005, p. 78).

Thus, the psychoanalytic method would consist of making conscious what was unconscious, paying attention to failed acts, symptoms and other manifestations or shifts in the psychic register.

The transformation of unconscious material into conscious material, as proposed by psychoanalysis, also brings us back to Green's (1994) statement about the transformation involved in the writing process, since, for him: "writing means, in the first place, transforming. Making the non-representability of unconscious fantasy pass into the non-representability of writing" (GREEN, 1994, p. 25). This was also stated by Clarice herself, in a different way, as we have just emphasized. However, in Green's statement, we find the aspect of fantasy, which is deeply involved in the process of writing, reading and the construction of identity, so we will try to understand this concept better. Although the concept of fantasy is extremely complex and rich in approaches in psychoanalytic theory, our aim here is not to delve into its theorization, but rather to explore the spaces whose doors are opened to us by it.

1.2 Identity, fantasy and literary creation

Eduardo Leal Cunha (2000), in his article *Uma interrogagao psicanalitica das identidades (A psychoanalytic interrogation of identities),* points to the need for a demarcation of the concept of identity, due to the variety of meanings attributed to it by countless sciences, including anthropology, philosophy and sociology, among others. Focusing on his identity as a psychoanalyst, the author discusses the notion of identity in psychoanalysis. According to him, such a concept, even though it has a foreign presence in the psychoanalytic field, is absolutely necessary.

According to Cunha (2000), the frequent use of the term "identity" throughout Freud's work does not make it easy to define:

> Throughout his work, although he often seems intensely concerned with establishing precise definitions for some fundamental concepts, in general Freud seems less concerned with any kind of conceptual rigidity than with using the resources of the German language, all of them, to get as close as possible to his object of study (CUNHA, 2000, p. 211).

In this way, without looking for strict definitions, Cunha (2000) tried to follow the use of "identity" in Freud's writings and found that "both in our case and in the current use of the German term, when we speak of identity, we are carrying out an operation of recognition and affirming a singularity". (CUNHA, 2000, p. 215).

Apart from similarity, it also denotes a difference, something in the nature of the individual that guarantees recognition and uniqueness.

In 1895, in the *Project for a Scientific Psychology* (FREUD, 1996a), the father of psychoanalysis systematized the functioning of the mind, linking the notion of identity to the investment and disinvestment of ideas (or representations) in the search for the re-establishment of a primary experience of satisfaction, at which point, most likely, the reference was to the satisfaction of a physical need, such as thirst or hunger. In other words, the psychic recognition of a perception responsible for the experience of pleasure and the search for the re-establishment of this satisfaction would consist of a "state of identity". This primitive moment in the constitution of the subject and the primary mode of psychic functioning will be responsible for uniquely marking the unconscious system. Thus, in Freud's conception, this experience of satisfaction will create the space of the first desire, with decisive consequences for the development of the individual.

In his essay *Oedipus and Passion,* Hdlio Pellegrino (1987) discusses this primitive moment in the constitution of the subject. Unlike animals (biologically and ontologically able to live in their environment), human beings are born primitive and without the necessary resources to deal with the experience of reality, so they have to develop them.

Biologically incomplete and premature, the human being receives, at birth, an excess of stimuli and excitements that it doesn't know how to deal with and, for lack of instinctive equipment, falls into an abyss, experiencing reality сото anguish. Faced with a reality that doesn't welcome it, the child retreats, seeking shelter in the past, taking refuge in a "fantasized" womb and denying birth - reality. "The child, at birth, is born out of anguish. It returns to the primordial house, the model of which is engraved in its mind" (PELEGRINO, 1987, p. 318). Faced with the anguish of reality, the child's first step will be to deny reality and take imaginary refuge in intrauterine life. In the words of
Pellegrino (1987):

> She creates for herself an enveloping and protective *sleeping bag,* where she is welcomed - and collected - in transit. Of course, the exchange with reality, from an objective point of view, is incessant. Into the darkness of the pretended womb where she shelters, the rivers of milk and honey of maternal care flow ceaselessly, inscribing the first - and immortal - experiences of satisfaction in the infant's psyche. These are the primordial lights in the darkness of the mind. They are flashes of pleasure that prefigure reality - and anticipate it. Life, in its essence, is a dream. We gradually grow from the imaginary dream to the symbolic dream, which, in its order, includes the imaginary and the real and transmits them through language (p. 318).

In this excerpt, Pellegrino reiterates Freud's assertion that the first motherly care will provide the infant with their first experiences of satisfaction, which are immortal as they will unconsciously mark the subject's mind, leading them to seek to re-establish these experiences and the pleasure they bring.

In this first moment, the child keeps inside everything that is useful, from the point of view of pleasure, and projects out everything that is bad or indifferent. Because she can't bear to part with the objects that fulfill her desires, she hallucinates them in her internal world and invests them according to the rhythm of her needs. In other words, at first, experiences of satisfaction will be represented hallucinatorily, for example: if I'm hungry, I start to hallucinate a breast capable of satisfying and placating it. In this sense, in the primitive psyche, the need appears in the form of satisfaction and dreams will serve to fulfill these desires, even though they are repressed. Pellegrino (1987) goes on to say that:

> Real experiences are, for the child, the stuff of dreams, just as clay is, for the sculptor, the stuff of work. There is no sculpture without clay, just as there are no hallucinatorily gratifying objects if there is no satisfying experience whose substance is reality, (p. 319).

However, the child begins to realize that the objects capable of satisfying them transcend his ability to create them, they have a life of their own, they are absent, they separate, leading him to realize that he doesn't have control over everything. At this point, the principle of reality comes into effect and "external objects begin to appear, in their alteritarian objectivity. The child has to accept them and make them *objects of desire,* replacing the internal, fantasized objects". (PELLEGRINO, 1987, p. 322).

Desire is thus characterized by the reinvestment of the mark left in the unconscious, by the original perception whose constant motor is the drive[1] , a force impossible to appease, responsible for setting the psychic apparatus in motion, making it desire. The concept of drive becomes fundamental to the discussion of the process of identity formation and subjective inscription; and, because of this, it will be further discussed in a later chapter of the work.

For now, it is important to understand that reliving satisfaction through hallucinatory means is not entirely satisfactory, as the way the psyche works will redirect towards motility, i.e. "desire begins to act in the field of the pre-conscious/conscious system and identity begins

'According to the *Dictionary of Psychoanalysis* (1998), the term pulse appeared in France in 1625, derived from the Latin *pulsio,* to designate the act of driving. Used by Sigmund Freud from 1905 onwards, it became a major concept of psychoanalytic doctrine, defined as the energetic charge found in the motor activity of the organism and in the unconscious psychic functioning of man. However, the concept underwent changes throughout Freudian theory and, because of this and its complexity, will be explored in greater depth later in this work.

to circulate above all in the field of thought rather than perception." (CUNHA, 2000, p. 10). In this context, fantasies are engendered, bringing together subject and reality, desire and object. According to Cunha (2000):

> It is in this private field of fiction that the subject gradually constructs his singularity, using the matrices provided by the others with whom he identifies - those who provide the words and affection necessary for him to experience different positions within the same intersubjective plot. (p. 16).

The constitution of identity is thus understood to be a game between impulses and the demands of the external world, a confrontation between the subject and otherness. The processes of the search for identity are glimpsed as the way in which the subject seeks order and circulation of his desire in the world. In this search, the individual locates the territory of fantasies as a privileged space for identities, insofar as fantasies are understood as the fulfillment of desires, albeit not always conscious ones.

Extremely interested in the examination of fantasies, Sigmund Freud gave a lecture on December 6, 1907, on the subject of *creative writers and daydreams.* For the father of psychoanalysis, the literary work is a substitute for childhood play, in that we are unable to give up the pleasure and satisfaction acquired from this activity, we just exchange it for another, forming a socially "more acceptable" substitute. In his words: "The writer softens the character of his egoistic daydreams by means of alterations and disguises, and bribes us with the purely formal, i.e. static, pleasure he offers us in the presentation of his fantasies." (FREUD, 1996c, p. 142).

We therefore ask ourselves: what are the possible types of alterations and disguises used by the writer; what characterizes such an aesthetic; how can the act of literary writing contribute to understanding the process of forming fantasies, recognizing the desires that surround them and, consequently, the way in which these desires are revealed, governing, singularizing and, why not, constituting a personal identity?

For Andre Green (1994), the literary text and the dream text have one thing in common: both are presented through secondary elaboration. In this way, fantasies are similar to literary texts, both mixing primary and secondary processes. Both processes, in trying to assume these secondary characteristics, occasionally leave traces of the primary processes on which they are based, due to the fact that they are forms of fiction. governed by desire. Therefore, the search for such traces in the Claricean text, chosen as the *corpus of* this research, will be one of the objectives of our study.

Furthermore, it's important to note that the traces left by the writer and the formal structure of his text also summon the reader to creative reverie, in other words, the text itself contains a potential for arousing fantasies that is actualized in the act of reading. Mijolla-Mellor, quoted by Moraes (2011, p. 76), says that "the fantasy that sustains the activity of writing is, consciously or not, that of contaminating the reader, of perverting him, or revealing to him the analogous impulses that will unravel in him during the reading". The reader is called upon by the writer to participate in the composition of the text's meanings precisely through their fantasies and impulses. And in this sense, Moraes (2011) suggests that we add to the literary creation of writing a literary creation of reading as well.

In this sense, we think that not only literary writing and the relationship between writer and text can provide us with elements to think about the process of fantasy production and identity construction, but also the reading process and the relationship between reader and text must be considered.

This fact invites us to think about and discuss the act of reading, and not just the creation of the text, both of which are inseparable from the humanizing influence of literature. Literary critic Antonio Candido (2004), considering literature to be a basic human right, as are the rights to food, health, housing, etc., refers to the humanizing role of literature, distinguishing three possibilities:

> (1) it is the construction of autonomous objects coro structure and meaning; (2) it is a form of expression, that is, it manifests the communities and worldviews of individuals and groups; (3) it is a form of knowledge, including diffuse and unconscious incorporation (CANDIDO, 2004, p. 176).

In other words, the literary work is characterized as a construction, with an organizing function to the extent that its character as an "organized thing" plays an ordering role in our own minds and feelings.

Still in the literary field, Goulart (2012) describes art, specifically literary writing, as one of the means found by human beings to confront the existential anguish resulting from not knowing their own identity. In other words, literature is also the result of the impossibility of answering the question: who am I?

On the basis of these statements, in this paper we seek to understand how Clarice Lispector's literary writing, specifically in the short stories in *The Beauty and the Beast,* provides us with elements to reflect on the human condition and its inherent complexity, especially with regard to the process of constructing identity[2] .

[2]The term identity, in the singular, is thus used in this work, starting from an outdated vision of a unified and stable subject, in order to enter into processes of deconstruction of this thought, both in psychoanalysis and in

1.3 Why Clarice?

The Freudian association between fantasy and literary creation is widespread, in other words, Freud believes that in every artistic manifestation it is possible to identify unconscious traces insofar as they all relate to the manifestation of desires. Among so many books, we have chosen Clarice Lispector's *Beauty and the Beast as* our object of study, and we will try to clarify some of the reasons that led us to this choice.

The father of psychoanalysis often turned to art in order to better elaborate his clinical constructions, making it clear that art precedes psychoanalysis. A Freudian position recalled by Lacan when he said: "With Freud and in his subject, the artist always precedes him and there is no way of doing psychology where the artist opens the way." (apud REGNAULT, 2001, p. 20). We share this thought and, although the chapters of this work begin with theoretical psychoanalytic arguments, it was Clarice's work that first aroused our curiosity about the construction of identity and then guided us *to* certain psychoanalytic discussions. We believe that bringing Lispector's writing closer to psychoanalysis can be an extremely fruitful encounter, mainly because the art of literary writing, here concretized in Clarice, can meet psychoanalysis in the place where conceptual organization comes up against the very limits of language.

Clarice's writing has a style that is difficult to grasp, averse and rebellious to names, revealing undiscovered aspects of language and, consequently, referring to something primitive and archaic in us. Her entry into Brazilian literature was impactful, representing a revolution in literature which until then had been represented by regionalist novels that portrayed social reality, forms of injustice and power relations. In this scenario, she began her career in 1943 with the publication of her first novel *Perto do Cororaqdo selvagem, the* title of which anticipates the visceral, sentimental and primitive aspects revealed in her writing.

Just as Freud was considered by many to be a transgressor, Clarice Lispector transgresses much of what was established as the benchmark for a novel and embarks on other paths, with another literary form, which doesn't have a linear presentation, secure finishes and well-defined characters. She goes to strange lands, to the tortuous and obscure paths of the unconscious, as she tells us in an excerpt from her novel *A Breath of Life* (Pulsagoes):

literature, and arrive at a notion of a fragmented post-modem subject; composed not of a single one, but of "various identities", sometimes contradictory or unresolved. In other words, throughout this work, we will also try to understand how identity becomes plural, mobile and continually transformed, in an infinite process in the relationship between the subject and the other.

> The danger of touching what is hidden - and the world isn't hidden, it's hidden in its roots submerged in the depths of the sea. To write I have to put myself in the void. It is in this void that I intuitively exist. But it's a terribly dangerous void: I draw blood from it. I'm a writer who is afraid of the trap of words: the words I say hide others - which ones? Maybe I'm saying them. Writing is a stone thrown into the deep end [...] That's how the book comes to me this time. (LISPECTOR, 1999b, p. 13;20).

This passage reinforces Freud's position on literary art, a pogo rich in depth, as well as the position we hold сото reference for our work.

Clarice Lispector's work is vast, rich in interpretations and literary criticism. However, the subject of our work takes us back to unknown, primitive forms, as well as to the bet on the new, on new forms of enunciation and subjectivation and, because of this, we chose to read *A bela e a fera* analytically precisely because it is one of the author's least studied and commented works, a work still unknown to many, which brings together everything from the first Claricean works to some of her last short stories.

A bela e a fera., published in 1979 by Nova Fronteira, is an organization of Clarice Lispector's short stories by Olga Borelli, a friend, collaborator and companion during the last years of the writer's life. The posthumous book brings together eight unpublished short stories, entitled *Historia interrompida, Gertrudes pede um conselho, Obsessao, O dehrio. The escape, Two more drunks. One less day* and *Beauty and the beast* or the *wound too big.* The first six stories are included in the first part of the book, as they were written by Clarice at the age of 20, still in the 1940s, and the other two were the last stories written by the author in 1977, the year of her death.

Nadia Gotlib (2009), in her book *Clarice - uma vida que se conta (Clarice - a life that is told),* reports that although the Pernambuco author's first published text was *O triunfo* - in the periodical *Pan, in* Rio de Janeiro, on May 25, 1940 - many other texts were written before this one, but were not published. Even though she began her activities as a novelist, Clarice wrote short stories, chronicles, among other ways of exchanging resources and ways of working with language. According to Gotlib (2009), while still at university, Clarice sent a volume of short stories to a competition run by the Josd Olympio bookshop and publishing house and, after finding out that she hadn't won the competition, discovered that they hadn't even received the original short stories, which had been lost along the way. According to Campos (1987), later, in 1950, Lispector said she had a copy of the short stories, but thought they were worthless. To this day, we don't know exactly what these stories were; however, there is a strong suspicion that they are the first six stories in the book *Beauty and the Beast.*

Assuming that these short stories really are, one wonders: were they really worthless?

The writer's improvement over the course of his practice is unquestionable; however, we have to consider that all of Clarice's work certainly arouses fascination and disquiet, even in the most naive reader. There's no way of tasting her words and coming away immune.

We believe that the short stories collected in *Beauty and the Beast, which have been* little studied in relation to the rest of the author's output, have not lost the strength and beauty of her texts. They can still provide us with rich elements for reflection, especially with regard to the human condition and its tireless search for an answer to the question: who am I?

Even though Clarice herself declared: "Don't worry about understanding. Living surpasses any understanding" (LISPECTOR, 1998a, back cover) her texts make it possible to "understand" ourselves...

In this work, we will seek, in particular, to understand more about the construction of identity in the relationship with the other, by analyzing the short stories in *Beauty and the Beast,* paying attention to the formal structure of the author's writing, as well as the effects it has on the reader.

These two directions - the writer's experiment and the reader's understanding - have been considered in Clarice's writing since it first appeared, as we can see in the statement by the critic Antonio Candido (1996), a novelty in the field of literature: "[...] it was a new experience, in both senses: the writer's experiment, the reader's understanding. [...] he was showing [...] that the world of the word is an infinite possibility of adventure, and that before being a narrated thing, the narrative is the form that narrates." (CANDIDO, 1996, p. XVIII).

The short stories in *Beauty and the Beast,* written at different times in the writer's life, also allow us to reflect on the formal variations in her writing, as well as on the many similarities that converge in Clarice Lispector's personal style.

In his book *O drama da linguagem - uma leitura de Clarice Lispector,* Benedito Nunes (1989) discusses Clarice's style, which, according to him, has a densely metaphorical expressive content, with "repetition as its longest-spectrum feature" (NUNES, 1989, p. 136). In other words, it is mainly through the reiteration of words that the author finds ways of giving emphasis, expressiveness and intensity to what she wishes to represent. In this global reading of Clarice Lispector, the author also states that in most short stories there is a single episode which serves as the core of the narrative, a moment of conflictive tension. "As the nucleus, i.e. the center of the epic continuity, such a moment of inner crisis appears differently conditioned and qualified depending on how the story develops." (NUNES, 1989, p. 84).

It's interesting to note that although Benedito Nunes didn't use the short stories from *Beauty and the Beast* in his analysis, the aforementioned characteristics are also present in the short stories. There is an inner crisis in the characters of the stories, with strong and polarized feelings, as well as a search for deeper reflection and ways of confronting the existential anguish of not knowing one's own identity. As the author states, "reflective acuity and restlessness form, in Clarice Lispector's characters, the inseparable links of 'self-consciousness'." (NUNES, 1989, p. 105).

In this tireless search for "self-awareness" and an authentic existence, the characters and also the narrator will repeatedly move through themes of birth, death, age, pain, joy, fear, loneliness, desire, anguish, speech, silence, nature, art, among others.

As an example of this search for self-awareness, which generates disquiet and also reflection, we cite here the questioning of the character Carla de Souza e Santos in the short story *A bela e a fera* ou *a ferida grande demais* (analyzed later in the work), which is narrated as follows: "She was... [...] Without comment, especially because the question lasted for a second: the question and the answer hadn't been thoughts in the head, they were in the body". [...] After all, who was she? [...] No comment, especially since the question lasted an instant: question and answer hadn't been thoughts of the head, they were of the body." (LISPECTOR, 1979, p. 142).

From this passage, we think that the search for authentic existence and the answer to the question "who am I?" become unattainable goals, as is the impossibility of language fully grasping reality. Being and saying, or writing, are thus equivalent to the extent of their impossibility.

Aware of this impossibility which, of course, affects the concept of identity and even makes it difficult to examine its representation in literary art, we will stick to what is possible to say and think, respecting the limits, but also trying to open up new possibilities for study and reflection on the subject.

1.4 O that the tales tell us

As we mentioned above, science and scientific concepts come up against many limits, including, fundamentally, language, and art can perhaps help us to overcome these limits. This is what Freud seems to have thought, as he made so much use of literature throughout his theorizing. Among them, we can find articles by Freud using literature as an interlocutor and as an object, providing us with important elements for observation and analysis, as we can read in *The Stranger* (1996f).

In this article, Freud tries to go beyond the more obvious association of the strange with the unfamiliar. It is based on a linguistic ambiguity, concretized in the etymology, formation of the abstract German noun *Unheimliche* (= strangeness) which, derived from *Heimlich.* which means familiar, to which the addition of the negative prefix *un comes to* mean o that which is unfamiliar and also something secret and hidden. Thus, in *unheimlich,* "[...] two sets of ideas stand out which, without being contradictory, are nevertheless very different: on the one hand it means o that which is familiar and pleasant and, on the other, o that which is hidden and kept out of sight." (FREUD, 1996f, p. 243). According to the psychoanalyst, not everything that is frightening or sinister evokes the feeling of strangeness, but only those situations in which the law of repression is also subverted, causing what should have remained "secret and hidden" to come to the surface. In other words, the stranger derives his terror not from some external or unknown source, but, on the contrary, from something strangely familiar that overcomes any efforts on the part of the individual to separate himself from it.

We can see in the texts of *Beauty and the Beast* the presence of epiphanic moments, of an encounter with something common, familiar, *heimlich,* which, dialectically, is transformed into its *unheimlich* opposite, causing many narratives to be divided into two moments: one before the encounter with the strange, unsettling thing, and one after.

We think that the encounter with the *familiar stranger* evokes helplessness and causes the character to plunge into a moment of epiphany. In addition, the sensation of "strangeness" and unease, in the contact with something familiar that should have been kept hidden, but came to light, can also be felt by the reader, and this feeling is responsible for a multiplicity of analytical interpretations of the text. In this sense, we will describe our observations of the characters' disturbing encounter with the *stranger,* as well as the strangeness felt while reading the texts.

The short story *Gertrudes Asks for Advice* tells the story of a teenage girl called Gertrudes, whose nickname is Tuda, who, at the age of seventeen, asks for help, through letters, from a female advisor and writer - a contributor to a magazine:

> The worst thing was that he only remembered the letter he had sent. "Ma'am, I'm seventeen and I wanted to..." Idiot, absolutely idiot. "I'm tired of moving around. Sometimes I can't sleep, even because my sisters sleep in the same room and move around a lot. But I can't sleep because I keep thinking about things. I've already decided to commit suicide, but I don't want to anymore. Can you help me? (LISPECTOR, 1979, p. 25).

The teenager seems to write to the counsellor in an attempt to rid herself of the "incommunicability" and state of isolation towards which she is heading, thus seeking a kind of identity with the world around her, which seems strange and distant.

After sending many letters, the doctor proposed a meeting: "Until the doctor ended up writing to her, calling her into the office." (LISPECTOR, 1979, p. 26). There will then be a meeting between the two characters, also narrated by this narrator who is sometimes external and omniscient, and sometimes merges with the consciousness of these characters, also making us reflect on the complexity of the process of constructing the identity of a subject who often merges with another. This is one of the first aspects we're interested in highlighting: the narrative form of the short story, in other words, observing the narrator who is sometimes external, sometimes confused with the protagonist's consciousness, leading the reader to "flit" between the spheres: internal and external, inside and outside, conscious and unconscious. Let's see:

> **Outside, everything was very nice.** I could see the roofs of the houses, the red flowers in a window, the yellow sun pouring down on everything. There was no better time than two in the afternoon.
> I didn't want to wait because I'd be afraid. And then I wouldn't give the doctor the impression I wanted to make. **Don't think about the interview, don't think. Quickly invent a story, tell a thousand, remember the good things** (LISPECTOR, 1979, p. 25, emphasis added).

What stands out in this passage is the narrator's take on the character in free indirect speech, and also the movement of his narrative which, after describing an external environment, seems to internalize and thus expose a stream of consciousness of the character Gertrudes, her anxiety and her fear of meeting the counsellor.

We note that the meeting with the counselor was made possible after the character Gertrudes sent the letters. It's interesting to note the means found by the teenager who, experiencing a lack of communication with the outside world, feeling that "there was no **correspondence** for her in the world", seeks a meeting through **correspondence.** In this double entry, we notice the polysemy, which makes use of the ambiguity of the term "correspondence", which, according to the *Aurelio Dictionary* (2010), means: "1. act or effect of corresponding. 2. exchange of messages by letters, telegrams, etc. 3. set of letters that an individual receives or sends. 4. rule by which each element of a set is associated with one or more elements of another." (p. 203). A1ëт that, from an etymological point of view, co + respondencia = a parallel speech to, companion and correspondence letter. O which emphasizes, even more, the "double" search of the character Gertrudes, who yearns not only for communication, but for an identification with this doctor.

This incommunicability with the external environment, emphasized and "doubled" by the work with language, seems to be related precisely to an alienation from the people around the teenager, an ignorance of internal "things". The narrator describes this external environment:

> But it's impossible to be big in a coто o sen environment. They interrupted her with the most banal remarks: "Have you showered, Tuda?" Or, if not, the look on the faces of the people at home. A simple, distracted look, completely oblivious to the noble fire burning inside her. Who could persist, she thought angrily, in such vulgarity? (LISPECTOR, 1979, p. 28).

The character didn't seem to find answers to the fire burning inside her, often "biologicist" answers, like those of her parents:

> Her mother, for example, didn't like her going out at night, claiming that it was too hot. She had to have her throat operated on and she always had a cold. But her father told her that there is good in evil and that tonsils were a defense for the body. And also, what nature had created had its function. (LISPECTOR, 1979, p. 30).

If, as her father believed, "what nature had created had its function", Tuda wondered what her function was; what her role was? She wanted to ask the counselor: "What do I do with myself? But she couldn't sum up her state in that question." (LISPECTOR, 1979, p. 31).

Faced with this question, she daydreamed of a freedom of fulfillment possible only in her fantasies and daydreams. She often imagined herself leading a crowd of men and women to worship her, saving the poor, or being a nurse, saving lives, wishing for different eyes from those distracted and oblivious to the fire that burned inside her. That's why she imagined that the counselor would have "strong eyes", capable of understanding her.

However, the encounter with this other woman was different from what she had dreamed. The counselor's lipstick, smudged off her lips in an attempt to be sensual, her vacant stare, as well as other "strangenesses", made Gertrude want to run away, especially after the doctor's explanation, which seemed similar to that of her parents:

> - Everything you feel is more or less normal, it will pass. You're intelligent and you'll understand what I'm going to explain to you. Puberty brings disturbances and...
> No, Doctor, what a shame. She was already too big for such things, what she felt was more beautiful and even...
> - This will pass. You don't have to work or do anything extraordinary. If you want to - she was going to use her old "truc" and smiled - if you want to get a boyfriend. So...
> She was just like Amelia, Lidia, everyone, everyone! (LISPECTOR, 1979, p. 31).

We see here the indignation of the character Gertrudes at the generalist explanation of the doctor, whose advice resembles self-help psychology, whose "truc", in an ironic tone in the narrative, denounces a disregard for the singularity of the subject.

Similar restlessness, and even indignation, can also be seen in another character in the same book, Elvira, the protagonist of the short story *A fuga.*

The short story *Escape* tells of a day when the character Elvira, tired of her routine life, leaves home on a cloudy day, breaking away from her usual life for a few moments and constructing another imaginary reality. It's interesting to note that the description of the external scenery, the cloudy day announcing the heavy rain that will fall next, seems to correspond to the internal scenery that is emerging in the character, which is what frightens her the most. Let's see:

> It started to get dark and she was afraid. The rain was falling steadily and the pavements shone wetly in the light of the lamps. People with umbrellas and raincoats were rushing past, their faces tired. [...] I wanted to sit on a bench in the garden, because I didn't really feel the rain and didn't mind the cold. Just a little afraid, because she hadn't yet decided which way to go. (LISPECTOR, 1979, p. 99).

The path mentioned above, when referring to the direction the character would take soon after in her journey, metaphorizes her desire to take another path in her life, a desire for other choices and attitudes. The reader can thus interpret, considering the staging of the character's daydreams in the text.

Elvira's first daydream was that she had left home and would never go back: "Now that she had decided to leave, everything was reborn. [...] She had been married for twelve years and three hours of freedom restored her almost entirely to herself: - the first thing to do was to see if things still existed." (LISPECTOR, 1979, p. 100).

Through the character's daydreams, we get to know her reality, her boring routine and the extent to which her imagination enjoyed a freedom that she didn't experience in her day-to-day life; on the contrary, she experienced an imprisoning marital relationship. Elvira's husband seems to represent a rational, repressive and controlling society, with which she doesn't identify:

> Desires are ghosts that fade away as soon as you turn on the lamp of common sense. Why do husbands have common sense? It's because they're particularly solid, good and never make mistakes. Of the people who only use one brand of pencil and say by heart what is written on the sole of their shoes. You can ask him without fear what the train timetable is, what the busiest time of day is and even in which region of the globe monkeys reproduce most quickly. (LISPECTOR, 1979, p. 101-102).

Elvira's thoughts and daydreams are permeated by social and marital questions, as well as desires for change, transgression and escape, involving situations in which there is no limit and no support, for example, the image of the subject who was not subject to the law of gravity, which she had fantasized about since she was a child:

> In the chapter on the force of gravity, in primary school, he had invented a man with a bent dock. The force of gravity didn't work on him... So he fell off the earth, and he kept falling, because the earth didn't know where he was going. Fall where? Then he'd figure it out: he'd keep falling, falling and he'd get used to it, he'd even eat falling, sleep falling, live falling, until he died. And would he keep falling? But at that moment, the man's agreement didn't distress her; on the contrary, it brought her a taste of freedom she hadn't felt for years. Because her husband had a unique property: his presence was enough to stop the slightest movement of her thoughts (LISPECTOR, 1979, p. 101).

The imprisonment of marriage and her husband's repression seem to be the facts that most distress and unsettle the character, leading her to imaginatively construct another reality: "[...] I was a married woman and now I am a woman" (LISPECTOR, 1979, p.102). However, she lacks the courage to truly break with material reality; the protagonist ends up returning to her home and to life alongside her husband.

The scenario of an imprisoning marriage and an external environment full of social repression, accompanied by a strong questioning of the female character and protagonist, is also seen in another short story from the same book: *Obsession.*

The short story *Obsessao,* among the eight stories found in *A bela e a fera*, is considered to be the most studied and commented on by critics, who, for the most part, draw attention to the slowness of the plot and some formal aspects considered questionable, while at the same time highlighting the presence of some tendencies that would become established in Clarice Lispector's writing. Since the short story dates from 1941, it belongs to the group of short stories from the writer's youth and presents us with an experimental narrative that makes use of various resources that will be taken up and reworked in more mature writing; there is also the presence of embryos of themes that will recur in the author's future works.

To analyze the short story, we will use the study by Yudith Rosenbaum (1997), which highlights the traces of perversity and sadism in Clarice Lispector's writing, and also the research by Jane Pinheiro de Freitas (2002), whose main focus is to show the anticipation of important aspects of the author's writing in her first short stories grouped together in the book *Beauty and the Beast.* Also paying attention to the anticipation of important aspects in the author's writing, in relation to the short story *Obsession,* Rosenbaum says: "[...] the seeds of the concerns most dear to the author are already visible, especially the work with tension and conflict, the reminiscent approach, the mimetic language of subtleties and emotional nuances and [...] the perverse play in love relationships [...]" (ROSENBAUM, 1997, p. 240).

With regard to tension and conflict, we can see that the tone of the narrative begins peacefully and gradually becomes tense until it returns to its previous resting place, which is related to the psychological state of the narrator at the time of the story. The story is narrated in the first person, by the protagonist named Cristina, who is trying to recall her experience of getting involved with a man called Daniel, in an attempt to find meaning in her story, a meaning that can be rescued through words.

The character Cristina is willing to tell us about her experience because she needs to understand it better and, by clarifying aspects for herself, she provides understanding where there was previously ignorance, while at the same time inviting us to join her in investigating the process of transformation that will take place within the inner self. In the words of Freitas (2002), "[...] Cristina is the sole mediator between the narrated world and the supposed reader interlocutor to whom she tells her adventure of searching for the self through otherness." (p. 60).

When we said that the tone of Cristina's narrative begins peacefully and gradually deepens until it returns to its previous repose, we wanted to point out the psychological state of the character, who initially experiences a tranquillity related to her surroundings; this tranquillity, however, is tormented as she comes into contact with her inner, primitive and unconscious aspects, through her encounter with the character Daniel.

In the first moment of the narrative, Cristina describes her restrained childhood, the tranquillity of a comfortable and superficial life, before meeting Daniel:

> I was born to simple people, instructed by the wisdom that comes from experience and common sense. From my childhood until I was fourteen, we lived in a nice house in the suburbs, where I studied, played and moved around carefree under the benevolent gaze of my parents. (LISPECTOR, 1979, p. 43)

Although she describes the peaceful and conflict-free environment in which she lived, the protagonist points out her dependence on the gaze of others and the foreshadowing of the "sad fruits" that would blossom in this land, since even though she lived a simple life, but without material difficulties, she often found herself in a state of anguish and melancholy. He reports:

> At times, causeless melancholy darkened my face, a warm and incomprehensible longing for times never lived before inhabited me. Not at all romantic, I immediately dismissed it as a useless feeling that doesn't connect with the really important things. Which things? She didn't define them well and included them in the ambiguous expression "things of life". (LISPECTOR, 1979, p.45).

Even though it was still incomprehensible, this melancholy was something latent within Cristina. According to Freitas (2002), it was:

> [...] a melancholy that didn't come to the surface, perhaps because the path to this intimate place, the place where the secrets lay, was still part of the unknown. The "warm longing" was not for what she had experienced, but for what she had yet to experience, for something that could give her a life beyond the restricted world she knew (p. 47).

The family organization and "warmth" in which Cristina found herself was only shaken by events capable of "disturbing the soul", such as birth, marriage and death. The protagonist, como "just any young girl", had dreams of getting married, having children and "finally being happy", and so she marries Jaime at the age of 19, a man with a fiery temperament whom she considered como an extension of her parents and her previous home. Up to a certain point in the narrative, Cristina's behaviour is described within the model for which the Brazilian woman of the 1940s was destined: to be restrained, a good wife, contributing to her husband's success and organizing the household. The protagonist's life revolved around the four walls that sustained her world: "Jaime. Me. Home. Mama". However, Cristina's vague restlessness is a sign that the social mask has been broken and she won't remain in the calm that marked her days. Little by little, disagreements with family conventions, restlessness and feelings of apathy began to emerge:

> I notice now that a certain apathy, rather than peace, has grayed my actions and my desires. I remember that Jaime had once said to me, a little emotionally:
> - If we had a child...
> I replied, inattentively:
> - What for6
> Denso ven isolated me from the world, and without knowing it, an abyss distanced me from myself (LISPECTOR, 1979, p. 46).

However, Cristina's detachment from herself and the anguish-desire within her are extemalized in the illness she acquires: typhoid fever. Even after she has recovered from the serious illness, her soul remains convalescent and her illness will be the trigger for her trip to Belo Horizonte. The illness prompts her to reflect, a state that will lead her inward, enabling her to come closer to self-knowledge.

The decision to travel to Belo Horizonte is taken by the family, but it will be the protagonist's first moment of freedom. This freedom, as is usually the case with Clarice's characters, is transformed into unease. Let's see:

> And one day, when I had already forgotten my "convalescent" attitude, they told me that I would be spending two months in Belo Horizonte, where the good climate and the new environment would strengthen me. There was no approval. Jaime took me

> there on a late train. He got me a good pension and left, leaving me alone, with nothing to do, suddenly thrown into a freedom I hadn't asked for and didn't know how to use (LISPECTOR, 1979, p. 46).

This nocturnal journey, which also allows us to think about the journey into the unknown, takes the character to a boarding house in the city, where she finds herself alone for the first time. Cristina describes how she felt: "What had sustained me until then were not convictions, but the people who had them. For the first time, they were giving me a chance to see with my own eyes. For the first time they were isolating me from myself." (LISPECTOR, 1979, p. 47).

It will be in this context that the narrator will meet Daniel, also a guest at the same hostel where she will be staying. The encounter with this other and the consequent shock for the character will not happen through seeing (as is the case with many of Clarice Lispector's characters), but mainly through listening, since the protagonist is attracted by a conversation between Daniel and another guest. Listening to the conversation immediately makes Cristina aware of Daniel's disregard for the established, and that's enough for her to find herself attracted to him - he's precisely the opposite of her; he's her antithesis, her antagonism, at least apparently and at first:

> And I was surprised and amused: I'd never heard anyone rebel against work, "such a serious obligation". Jaime's or Dad's rebellion at most only took the form of a lament, of no importance. In general, I had never thought that it was possible not to accept, to choose, to rebel... (LISPECTOR, 1979, p. 49).

At the same time as she felt strongly attracted to what Daniel represented, the narrator tried to avoid him, coто if she wanted to defend her amorphous life from anything that might disturb her comfort. But she herself says: "It was in vain. Daniel was the danger. And towards him I was walking". (LISPECTOR, 1979, p. 49).

Cristina's attraction to Daniel will intensify even more when she hears a maxim repeated by him in one of his seductive dialogues: "Accomplishments kill desire - said Daniel." (LISPECTOR, 1979, p. 50). Daniel's words bring Cristina into contact with the primacy of desire, of her previously unknown desires, especially the desire to search for this unknown self.

The male character seemed to notice Cristina's attraction and, above all, the way she positioned herself in relation to the "things of life", in such an opposite way to him. He would then ask her questions that embarrassed her, such as: "- Cristina, do you know that you live?

[...] - Cristina, is it good to be unconscious? [...] - Cristina, you don't want anything, do you? [Cristina, do you want me to wake you up?" (LISPECTOR, 1979, p. 58).

Daniel's questions and conversations with him awakened inner aspects in Cristina that had been dormant for a long time:

> Yet it was the truth. Me, so simple and primitive that I had never wanted anything with intensity. Me, unconscious and joyful, "because I had a joyful body"... Suddenly, I woke up: what a dark life I'd had until then. Now... now I was reborn. Vividly, in pain, in that pain that slept quietly and blindly in the depths of myself (LISPECTOR, 1979, p. 60).

Unlike the well-known fables, in which the princess is awakened by a prince and they both have a happily ever after, in *Obsession,* the protagonist is "awakened" by this man, who, in his description, is more like a beast than a prince, and they both begin to reflect and get in touch with the most painful aspects of life and of themselves.

Despite her suffering, the narrator prefers to get in touch with the depths of her desire rather than remain in her previous "blissful blindness". She calls this process of rediscovering herself "transformation". For now, it's important to emphasize that the narrator's transformation came about through the discovery of intimate and hitherto unconscious aspects related to desire. As she describes сото: "And the greatest harm that Daniel did to me was to awaken in myself that desire which is latent in all of us. In some people it just wakes them up and poisons them, as in my case and Daniel's. For others it leads to laboratories, journeys, absurd experiments, adventure. Madness." (LISPECTOR, 1979, p. 57).

These countless paths taken towards desire, to which Cristina refers, will also be represented in other characters in the work - for them, Freud reserved the concept of sublimation, as will be seen below.

Furthermore, with regard to the process of inner transformation, we are also led to think about the function of the book - just as сото Daniel awakened questions and feelings within Cristina, he is also capable of doing so within the reader. There's no doubt that, for a long time in history, the effects of reading could be described from the point of view of impregnating and poisoning the reader. It's no wonder that, in order to maintain the power of the state, the great dictators also limited the scope of reading. Nazi propaganda, for example, included images of the burning of books in Berlin in 1933. On the occasion, an enthusiastic crowd was fooled by the censors' speech: "Against the exacerbation of unconscious impulses based on the destructive analysis of the psyche, for the nobility of the human soul, I give the works of Sigmund Freud to the flames - declaimed one of the censors before burning Freud's books."

(MANGUEL, 1997, p. 316).

Like Freud's books, many others went up in flames, with literature placed in opposition to morality and alongside transgression and sin, possessing the ability to contaminate the reader's mind and awaken unconscious impulses.

Returning to *Beauty and the Beast,* another character who is "awakened" to aspects that were previously hidden, following an encounter with another character is Carla de Souza e Santos, a madam from Rio *and the* protagonist of the short story *Beauty and the Beast or Being Too Big.*

The short story tells, in the third person, the experience of a woman called Carla de Souza e Santos, a madam from Rio de Janeiro, who, on leaving the lobby of the Copacabana Palace hotel, has to wait for her chauffeur to come and stands in the street. At that moment, she felt like she was enjoying herself for the first time in her life: "She couldn't remember when she had last been alone with herself. Perhaps never. It was always her - with others, and in those others she reflected herself and the others reflected her. Nothing was pure, she thought without understanding herself." (LISPECTOR, 1979, p. 133).

The protagonist's thoughts seemed tranquil until the moment a beggar approached her to ask for money; her tranquillity was abruptly interrupted by the sight of a huge wound on the beggar's leg: "'Help!!!' she shouted to herself as she saw the huge wound on the man's leg. 'Help me, God,' she said softly (LISPECTOR, 1979, p. 135). From that moment on, the beggar's wound became a mirror in which Carla saw herself reflected: "She - the others. But death doesn't separate us," she suddenly thought, and her face took on the look of a mask of beauty, and not the beauty of people: her face hardened for a moment." (LISPECTOR, 1979, p. 135).

Used to driving around in a car, going to lavish parties and having contact with people only from her "milieu", she feels the impact of this encounter with the other, with the different. At first, she remembers her comfortable, soft life "like a cat's leap", she remembers her banker husband, her well-dressed friends, her frequent preoccupation with beauty and the security that the traditions of her environment brought her: "Beauty can lead to the kind of madness that is passion. She thought: "I'm married, I have three children, I'm safe". (LISPCETOR, 1979, p. 134).

However, the sight of the beggar's wound in the encounter with this other marks an epiphanic moment in the protagonist's life, as it makes it possible to lay bare many things: "[...] then she began to look inside herself and things really began to happen." (LISPECTOR, 1979, p. 138).

In a process of identification and "disidentification" with the beggar, Carla then begins to question traditions and the way the world works, thus positioning herself as a subject in the face of these questions and reflects: "And the essential magic of living - where was it now? In what corner of the world? In the man sitting on the corner? Is the spring of the world money? [...]" However, the text continues: "But he wanted to pretend that it wasn't. She felt so, so rich that she felt sick." (LISPECTOR, 1979, p. 143).

Let's remember that the tone of this short story is extremely similar to another short story by the same author: *Amor,* published in (1964) in the book *Legiao Estrangeira. Amor is* a third-person account of the day of a woman called Ana, a housewife who, while out shopping on a streetcar, is surprised by the sight of a blind man chewing gum. The sight of this blind man has an impact on the character, causing ambiguous feelings, previously dormant, to rise to the surface, triggering in the protagonist an eruption of self-awareness and reality. Let's read it to remember:

> She had calmed life down so well, had taken such care that it didn't explode. She kept everything in serene understanding, separated one person from another, clothes were clearly made to be worn and you could choose from the evening movie - everything was done so that one day followed another. And a blind man chewing gum highlighted it all. And through pity, a life full of sweet nausea appeared to Ana, right up to her mouth (LISPECTOR, 1994, p. 34).

We have identified, then, the point of greatest similarity between the short stories mentioned, that alterity exerts a disturbing influence on the stability that previously existed in the lives of the characters - Clarice Lispector's subjects. This is an extremely important aspect in the process of constructing identity, and one that we have insisted on in this research.

Despite the restlessness and discomfort generated by the force of otherness, we also notice great torment in the absence of otherness, in other words, when the other is absent or becomes unattainable. This can be identified in the short story *Two more drunks.*

The short story *Mais dois bebados is* narrated in the first person by the protagonist, who has no home of his own and finds himself in a state of profound loneliness. Although, for him, solitude is "too strong a drink" (LISPECTOR, 1979, p. 108) and he seeks to drink from other sources, it is precisely solitude, the first that seems to make him more intoxicated.

Seeking to alleviate this empty and distressing state, the narrator walks from bar to bar, looking for someone with whom he can share his daydreams: "I looked for a man or a woman. But no one particularly appealed to me. They all seemed to be enough, spinning around in their own thoughts. No one needed me." (LISPECTOR, 1979, p. 109). For him, people were self-sufficient, unlike him, who felt a great need for others, even to recognize himself.

The protagonist, full of questions, feelings and emotions, is looking for a way to "spill a little before it overflows entirely" (LISPECTOR, 1979, p. 108), and in a new attempt to connect with the other, he makes a call to Emma:

> - Aid, Ema!
> - Oh dear, at this hour!
>
> I hung up. Was it a lie? The tone was real, the energy, the beauty, the love, that eagerness to give my excess were real. Only the phrase imagined so effortlessly was a lie (LISPECTOR, 1979, p. 108).

It's interesting to note that, not by chance, before "overflowing entirely", the protagonist imagines communicating with "Ema", the only name mentioned in the story, whose letters also bear the word "mother". This brings us back to the original helplessness of the recëт-born child who, as mentioned, is in a state of impulsive overflow with which he doesn't know how to cope and therefore depends on another to provide him with this initial support. This situation of original helplessness will mark the human condition and will be "relived or remembered" throughout life, in situations such as the loss of love, the loss of an object or experiences of separation.

The protagonist of the story seems to be experiencing a situation that evokes such helplessness and, since the communication he has achieved with Emma is only imaginary and therefore "incompletely satisfactory", he is led to look for other resources. He then starts a conversation with a stranger chosen from among countless other people: "I saw him. Just like everyone else. But so alike that he formed a type. This one, I decided, this one" (LISPECTOR, 1979, p. 109). Here, we refer to the Freudian theorizing set out at the beginning of this chapter, about the movement of the subject who, upon realizing the incomplete satisfaction obtained through internal and hallucinatory objects, seeks such satisfaction in external objects, thus turning them into objects of desire. In this case, after imagining a telephone conversation, the protagonist decides to choose a person from the place he was in to try to communicate with.

The conversation between them is lukewarm and the narrator is amazed at the insensitivity of this other person when he talks about his son's illness:

> - But you were talking about your son!
>
> He looked at me for a moment. Then he smiled:
>
> - Ah, yes. Well, he's in a bad way.
> - What's wrong with him?
> - Angina, the pharmacist said angina.
> - Who's the boy with?
> - With her mother.
> - And you don't stay with her?

- What for?
- Dear God... At least to suffer with her... O senhor e casado com a moca[9] (LISPECTOR, 1979, p. 109-110).

Faced with indifference towards his son's illness, the narrator then creates an imaginary scene in which the child dies and his body is eaten by rats, the same ones that will eat away at his mother's body, alone and passed out after the sad event. Describe the man:

> The child gasps, dying. Dying. His little head is bent, his eyes are open, fixed on the wall, obstinately. Everything is silent and the girl doesn't know what to do. The child has died and she's suddenly unoccupied. She falls on the bed, crying, tearing her clothes: "My son, my poor son! And death, and death!" The rats in the house get scared and start running around the room. They climb up her son's face, which is still warm, and gnaw on his little mouth. The woman screams and faints for two hours. The rats also visit her body, happily, quickly, their little teeth gnawing here and there (LISPECTOR, 1979, p. 110).

Despite the tragic speech, the narrator is disappointed to see that he hasn't aroused any emotion in the stranger; on the contrary, he's made the other man sleep: "His head lying on his arms, he didn't move. For a moment I was frightened. What if he was dead? I shook him and he raised his head, barely able to look at me with his sleepy eyes. I looked at him angrily." (LISPECTOR, 1979, p. 111). This difficulty of to get in touch with this other and the impossibility of communication, Freitas (2002) states that:

> [...] The protagonist is looking for someone in whom he can unveil himself, look inside himself, and into his own mysteries; but the other, seen as the way to unveil the self, won't let himself be discovered and remains unattainable, so the protagonist's resources become increasingly useless. (p. 33).

Indignant at the other's indifference, since "he should have thanked me for approaching him, because otherwise I would never have known he existed. Yet he persisted in his muteness, without even being moved by the opportunity to live" (LISPECTOR, 1979, p. 108), the narrator associates this behavior with a state of "ataraxia". *Ataraxiaë* a word of Greek origin that translates as "absence of restlessness", "tranquillity of mind", in other words, a state that is also unattainable for this man who is immersed in his restlessness and internal turbulence. At that moment, he is confronted with the difference between himself and the other: "But perhaps you don't understand: we are different. I suffer, in me the feelings are solidified, differentiated, already born with a label, conscious of themselves." (LISPECTOR, 1979, p. 112). The incommunicability between the two characters thus highlights a deeper conflict, between consciousness and unconsciousness, desire and non-desire, *ataraxia and* restlessness.

When, finally, a solution to these conflicts seems to emerge, and the strange interlocutor seems to speak, the narrative is abruptly interrupted: "Suddenly, he took the toothpick out of his mouth, his eyes blinking, his lips trembling as if he were going to cry, and he said:" (LISPECTOR, 1979, p. 114). This abrupt end to the narrative allows us to think of a state of unconsciousness on the part of the narrator himself, who, drunk, blurs the boundaries between consciousness and unconsciousness. In other words, in the short story *Two more drunks,* the narrative form and, above all, the abrupt break in the plot also "gets" the reader drunk, who, like the characters, is immersed in the malaise of the search for meaning.

Still with regard to the abrupt ending of the narrative, with the emptiness and silence that are repeated in Clarice's texts, we think that the reader has the power to speak, to offer his hands to build the text and to support the narrator who asks for his help. However, if the reader doesn't find support in the text, he also becomes helpless.

Inspired by the Freudian method, which considers written language to also be a space of unconscious production, we realize, then, through the analysis of these short stories, that the narrative forms tell us something beyond the content narrated. As Bellemin-Noel (1983) puts it:

> Let's just say here that we had to accept the idea of a different language, one that didn't just say, neither exactly nor truly, what it seemed to say. In the same way that the psyche did not constitute a kind of unified block with its suppositions and parts of competencies, the writing of the great works could not be equated with the transmission of a message with a single obvious meaning. Everyday words put together in a certain way acquire the power to suggest the unpredictable, the unknown; and writers are men who, by writing, speak, without knowing it, of things that literally "they don't know". (p. 12, emphasis added).

This quote by Bellemin-Noel (1983) sums up the idea that we have tried to develop throughout this first chapter: the decentering of the psyche and, consequently, the denial of a univocal identity, similar to the interpretation of a work, which can acquire multiple meanings.

We have seen, through the analysis, that the "hidden" meanings are being constructed from the reader's "strangeness" in the face of the "strangeness", gaps and silences in the text. In this sense, we once again turn to Birman's (2003) reflections, when he states that all the formations of the unconscious enunciated by Freud denote ways of being of the psyche, in which the self, in the cognitive register, literally fails in its instrumental functionality.
In other words:

> Both in the dream and in the failed act, in the lapse, in the joke and in the symptom, the "I" slips away from something that is momentarily deconstructed, showing the irruption of desire. [...] In short, imagination. coro excess and productive positivity,

> can then be highlighted, leaving the condition of negativity in which it was placed by classical psychology. (BIRMAN, 2003, p. 48).

In this way, all psychopathological disorders of the spirit would also come out of their condition of negativity and could be interpreted by the paradigm of the unconscious, insofar as they would be significant.

To endorse our reflection on psychopathological disorders and their condition of positivity or negativity, we turn to the short story *Delirium,* also found in *Beauty and the Beast.*

The story, in the third person, tells of the disconnected thoughts of a sick man in his bed, the content of which is often related to the creation of the planet, nature and death. It's not our job here to diagnose the character, but rather to observe how the contents of the delusions are exposed throughout the narrative and how they relate to the character's perception of himself and his surroundings.

The narrator of the story begins his narrative by describing the start of the sick man's day, from the moment he wakes up: "The day is high and strong when he gets up. He looks for his slippers under the bed, groping with his pds, while he snuggles into his flannel pajamas. The sun begins to cover the closet, reflecting on the floor the wide square of the window." (LISPECTOR, 1979, p. 85).

After describing the external environment with the arrival of the sun and daylight, the narrator merges his narrative with the protagonist's consciousness and enters his delirium:

> He shrinks down deeply, coто if it were raining outside, raining, and here some silent and silent braves would trap him and turn him into a small boy, small and dead. Dead. Oh, and o delirium... And o delirium. A very sweet light spreads over the Earth like a perfume. The moon slowly fades and a boyish sun shines down on the translucent braves... Fresh murmurs of pure water abandon themselves to the slopes. A pair of wings dances in the rosy atmosphere. Silencio, mens amigos. O diavai nascer. (LISPECTOR, 1979, p. 86).

In this way, the reader sees the birth of the day from another perspective, from the "delirious" perspective of this sick man. This mixture of narrative form also allows us to think about the mixture of the content of the delirium itself, which, Freud conjectured, is not a randomly formed content, but mixes the subject's external perceptions with internal and unconscious psychic contents. In this passage, the shrinking into a warm environment, together with the transformation "into a little boy, small and dead", refers us not only to the image of the fetus in fetal position inside the mother's womb, coто the idea of being "unborn", returning to the womb, the primordial home, coто reads in *Pellegrino.* This image allows us to think about the first movement of the subject who, at birth, faced with a distressing reality, takes refuge in the hallucinatory image of intrauterine life. We can also think of the ambiguity that surrounds the content of this delirium, which can refer to the birth of the day, but also to the birth of the character himself.

This ambiguous aspect of the delusions and of the narrative is also perceived at other moments in the story, for example, when a woman is approached, on whose wrist there was a watch, and the sick man understands that a dove is trapped. Let's see: "The hand tries to escape. He holds it back. It stays. The wrist. Thin and tender, it ticks. It's a dove he's trapped. The dove is frightened and its heart is ticking." In this passage we notice the sound play between "little pigeon" and "pulse", as well as the change in the rhythm of the narrative, strategies used by the author to confuse the reader too: the rhythm of the clock or the heartbeat of the imprisoned little pigeon?

It's important to note that the content of the protagonist's thoughts initially refers to the creation of planet Earth and then to its extermination. As he is ill and death is a clear threat, the sick man identifies with this fact, shifting it onto himself: "Help me, my land is withering... Then what will become of my light?" (LISPECTOR, 1979, p. 90). Planet Earth and character, light and life, are confused in the consciousness of the protagonist, who finds it difficult to distinguish between what refers to his delirium and what refers to reality: "- Ah, it's delirium. I'm sorry, in the end we don't know if it really happened or if it was a lie..." (LISPECTOR, 1979, p. 92).

In this way, the reader of this short story struggles to discriminate between what the text refers to as "reality" and what it describes as the content of the protagonist's delirium, finding himself immersed in the complexity of the human mind. We also conjecture that the ironic tone of the passage "Ah, the delirium", repeated countless times throughout the narrative, points to a criticism of the medical and perhaps psychiatric discourse, which rigidifies diagnoses.

At the end of the story, the psychological disturbance loses even more of its negative aspect and makes room for the positivity of imagination, as the protagonist transforms mental pain into prosthetic material:

> He straightens up in his chair, a little surprised, dazzled. A flurry of thoughts suddenly cross his mind... Yes, why not? Even with the brunette... Does the whole delirium appear before your eyes? Like a painting... Yes, yes... It cheers you up. But what poetic material it contains. "The Earth is having children" And the dance of the beings on the open wounds? The heat returns to his body in light waves.
>
> - "Do me a favor," he said eagerly, "call Mrs. Marta...
>
> She's coming.

> - Would you like to bring me a pencil that's on the table? And a pencil too... (LISPECTOR, 1979, p. 94).

In this excerpt we see once again that thoughts intertwine in the character's mind based on identifications, for example the identification he has with the planet Earth. The planet begets children, just as he "gives birth" in the process of creating the text.

After discussing "strangeness" throughout this chapter, we close by mentioning the possibility of light and the process of creation, in the desire to keep the flame of hope, curiosity and creativity burning throughout the writing of the work, as well as its reading.

2 FROM THE SELF TO THE OTHER

> *Before, I had wanted to be someone else in order to know what wasn't me.*
> *I understood then that I had already been the others and that was easy.*
> *My greatest experience would be to be the other of the others: and the other of the others was me (LISPECTOR, 1964, p.142).*

In the first chapter we discussed the first decentering, from a Freudian point of view, following the discovery of the unconscious, which consequently inaugurated the psychoanalytic method based on interpretation. Through this method, unconscious meaning would be constructed from formations of the unconscious, such as the symptom, the failed act, the fantasy, and would be revealed in the encounter with the other. According to Cunha (2005), this makes the model of psychoanalytic treatment itself paradigmatic:

> [...] in which the production of new meanings and subjective reordering take place not only in the suspension of the self that is produced in the patient with the method of free association, but above all in the encounter of this imaginative wandering with another suspension of the control of the self, which must take place in the analyst through floating action. It is in the paradoxical meeting of two absent selves that new meanings can become present. From this perspective, subjectivity needs to be taken not in its entirety, but as fragmented and dispersed, in all its potential (CUNHA, 2005, p. 80).

In this sense, the second movement in the deconstruction of the subject based on reason and consciousness shifted this subject from the self to the other, placing it outside of itself. This is why Birman (2003) states that the second deconstruction of the idea of the subject took place in the direction of the self to the other.

The analysis of fragments of some short stories from *Beauty and the Beast,* in the first chapter, already signaled an epiphanic aspect of the encounter between the self and the other, which would be replicated in the many encounters analyzed: of the teenager Gertrude with the counsellor; of Cristina with Daniel; of the Rio madam Carla de Souza e Santos and the beggar; of the reader with the literary text. These encounters enabled a deconstruction of the self through the exercise of intersubjectivity. However, the statements made from the analytical moments still lacked theoretical arguments to support the proposed interpretations; because of this, we will try to understand, with the help of psychoanalytic theory, the phenomena involved in the process of subjective transformation that takes place in the encounter between the self and the other.

Therefore, in this chapter, we will initially and briefly try to understand the movement of the second decentering of the idea of the subject pointed out by Birman (2003), in order to later understand how it can be represented in the literary text and become an operator of interpretative reading, with some caveats, of course - art far transcends the meanings that would be interpreted with psychoanalytic conceptual arguments, созо with any other operators of critical reading. And, as Candido (2004) rightly points out, the "organization" it makes possible of the chaos that precedes it goes beyond "explanations", searches for causes and projects itself into what Eco (2003) calls an "open work", open to a multiplicity of readings and interpretations.

Clarice Lispector's art is no different: the characters' constant search for the meaning of life and self-awareness, their striking encounter with the other or with what is different, the recurring theme of death, anguish and alienation, as well as a narrative structure full of voids and silences, invite the reader to question their own identity, participating in a process of deconstruction and reconstruction of the self in the intersubjective relationship with the text itself.

Ogden (1996), on the first page of his book *The Subjects of Psychoanalysis,* alerts the reader to the experience that will take place if he continues reading and allows us to think about the encounter between reader and text, as well as the experience of reading:

> The disturbing experience of being transformed into a subject you don't yet know, but recognize nonetheless [...] Reading is not simply a matter of examining, pondering or even testing the ideas and experiences presented by the writer. Reading implies a more intimate form of encounter. You, the reader, need to allow me to occupy you - your thoughts, your mind, since I have no other voice to speak but yours. If you intend to read this book, you need to give yourself the right to think my thoughts, while I need to allow myself to take your thoughts, so that neither of us will be able to claim o thought as our own exclusive creation. (OGDEN, 1996, p. 1).

The production of meanings resulting from a reading is not something exclusive to the reader, nor to the author, nor to the text alone, but, according to psychoanalytic interpretation, it becomes possible through the meeting of "two absent I's".

Let's think about Freud's formulations, which obviously didn't form on their own, they needed metaphors, models for identifying theoretical hypotheses, support to be said, and how much literature can be used by Freud, not only for this, but созо a model of discourse. There is a consensus among researchers that Freud's writing style is closer to creative writers than to the scientific-medical style of ëpoca, mainly because his writings, especially in clinical cases, were more like novels and came to constitute a literary style of their own. Sampaio (2005) states that it is "in the lineage of precursors and masters that we can understand the ascendancy of Literature over Psychoanalysis [...] we could say that Literature participates in the very birth of

Psychoanalysis." (p. 164). Extending the extent of the influence, according to this author, literature served as a model, object, auxiliary and rival to Freudian thought. As a model, literature was the parameter for Freud's approach to a novelistic narrative style; as an object, we recall an important Freudian text already cited in this dissertation, *The Stranger* (FREUD, 1996f), inspired by Hoffman's short story The *Man in the Sand (*1993). Literature also offered metaphors and participated in countless Freudian illustrations; and it is in the separation of what is art and what is science that we can find the Freudian distance from Literature, in an attempt to establish boundaries.

Considering all these places occupied, for Sampaio (2002), in relation to psychoanalysis, "literature appears as an **'other'**, in the precise sense of an adjunct to the constitution of an 'I'". (SAMPAIO, 2002, p. 153, emphasis added).

In order to further understand this function of the other, exercised by literature in relation to psychoanalysis, as well as the function of the other in the constitution of a self, the latter being the central aspect of our work, we will now delve into the elements involved in this relationship.

2.10 second decentering of the subject

The second Freudian decentering finds its fullest meaning with the introduction of the category "narcissism" in 1914. This is because, before elaborating the theory of narcissism, Freud thought of the "I" as a regulating instance, linked to reality and protected from the dissimulations of sexuality. Sexuality should be disciplined and put at the service of the conservation of the species, and the dualism of drive is characterized by the drive for conservation (drive of the self) *versus the* sexual drive.

However, following the discovery of the investment of libido[3] in the self and the object, Freud was led to reformulate his theory, and the self definitively lost its autonomy and sovereignty in the psyche. In this context, says Birman (2003):

> [...] the instance of the "I" also came to be conceived as sexualized, no longer directed solely by the disinterested search for truth. Therefore, the self would also be invested by the libido and would thus cease to have any transparency in its cognitive choices,

[3]According to the *Dictionary of Psychoanalysis,* by Elizabeth Roudinesco and Michel Pion (1998), the term libido is of Latin origin, translated as desire, and was initially used by sexology researchers to designate an energy proper to the sexual instinct. However, Sigmund Freud took up the term in an entirely different way, to designate the manifestation of the sexual drive in psychic life and, by extension, human sexuality in general. However, it is difficult to present a satisfactory notion of the concept of libido, since the theory of libido has evolved with the different stages of pulse theory, and the concept itself is far from having received a univocal notion.

> clouded as it would be by its erogenous demands, thus losing any neutrality in its reading of the world (p. 66).

Thus, the self that could previously, with its conservation impulses and its principle of reality, carry out cognitive operations in search of truth in a totally neutral way, is no longer totally neutral, since it is now also lost in a web of fantasies and desires, subject to the force of the impulse, dispersed and fragmented. Freud then deconstructs the idea of the stable unity of an ego, from its inception, by highlighting a long process of ego development, which requires external help.

As Freud says in his essay *'Narcissism: an introduction'.*

> [...] we are destined to assume that a unit comparable to the ego cannot exist in the individual from the very beginning; the ego has to be developed. The auto-erotic instincts, however, are there from the beginning, and it is therefore necessary for something to be added to auto-eroticism - a new psychic action - in order to provoke narcissism. (FREUD, 1996e, p. 84).

In other words, in these new Freudian formulations, the "I" would not be the original and totalizing instance of the psyche and the body, as previously thought, but derived from the investment of the other. Consequently, the ideals of integration, unity and permanence of identity become increasingly distant.

It would be the image of this privileged other that, in its narcissistic function, would invest libidinally in the self, placing it in an idealized place and, through a specular game, would make it possible to perceive its own body. Without the interference of this other, there would be no recognition or idealization of the self. We are referring here to what Freud called coto primary narcissism, in which all libido is directed towards the self, before being directed towards the object. O primary narcissism is characterized mainly by the child's choice of his or her person as the first object of love, in a stage preceding the full capacity to turn to external objects. In this first moment, the infantile narcissistic self is the ideal self, omnipotent and full, constructed imaginatively from the parents' narcissistic investment in the baby. Freud refers to the baby using the expression: "His Majesty the Baby." (FREUD, 1996e, p. 98). The psychoanalyst referred to the infant in this way after observing a painting from the Edwardian era, which bore this title and showed two London policemen interrupting heavy traffic to let a nanny cross the street pushing a child's baby carriage. He identified in that image, in the attitude of the policemen, a great similarity with the behavior of parents after the birth of a child, since, reliving their own narcissism, they overvalue the child, placing it at the center of all their concern, gaze and drive investment.

However, when faced with an ideal with which they have to compare themselves, an ideal derived from their parents, formed outside of them, imposed from outside and impossible to achieve, the child goes beyond the position of primary narcissism. This is the game of mirrors referred to by Jaqueline Moreira (2009), in her article *Revisiting the concept of the self in Freud: from identity to otherness.* According to her:

> [...] The ideal self is in the mirror image and not in the real child; there is an abyssal distance between the child and the ideas we think of. This double self can be called the narcissistic other. The child anchors itself in this image, constructs for itself this story of this dreamed-of place in the parents' desire, but it is necessary to abandon this position so as not to fall into the waters of death. (MOREIRA, 2009, p. 237).

The abandonment of this narcissistic position to which Moreira refers can be understood as an egoic split, a gap between the self and the ideal, causing the narcissistic formation of a substitute for the lost infantile narcissism, which Freud called the ideal of the self. The ideal of the self corresponds to secondary narcissism, the result of secondary identifications, the marks of abandoned object investments, implying the gradual abandonment of narcissistic omnipotence and the investment of the other сото otherness and difference.

This means that, initially, the image of this privileged other is necessary for the transformation of the fragmented body of autoeroticism into a unified and narcissistic body, in other words, narcissistic satisfaction is a necessary moment within libidinal life. However, in this context, the original self cannot distinguish the self from the other. The experience of castration[4] will be necessary for the self to have a special perception of otherness. As Moreira (2009) states, "the other is present from the start, but the self can only recognize otherness by contrasting it with its identity. Thus, the self only recognizes the dimensions of otherness after the encounter with the anguish of castration" (p. 239).

It is only after the experience of castration and, consequently, the recognition of the other's anteriority, i.e. the recognition of otherness, that the subject will be able to free themselves from the alienated image they have constructed.

Once again, we come across the complexity and ambiguity involved in the process of subjective constitution, in which the pain of separation opens up the possibility of recognizing otherness and inaugurates the hope of inscribing a self. The antagonisms involved in this

[4]Although the castration complex is considered extremely important in psychoanalytic theory, we won't go into depth in understanding this process, fearing that the scope it involves will distract us from the central focus of the work. For now, it's important to consider that Sigmund Freud called the castration complex the unconscious feeling of bitterness experienced by a child when it realizes the anatomical difference between the sexes.

process remind us of another work by Clarice Lispector, *Agua Viva,* specifically a letter written by the narrator, addressed to her love, and indicative of separation, in which she writes: "And with such profound joy. It's such hallelujah. Hallelujah, I cry out, a hallelujah that merges with the darkest human howl of the pain of separation but is a cry of diabolical happiness. Because no one holds me more." (LISPECTOR, 1998b, p. 9).

From this excerpt, we can see that the character weaves a vivid account of her subjectivity, alternating moments of deep anguish with others of renewed joy, based on the experience of separation from the other.

Similarly, we will continue our analysis of the tales in *Beauty and the Beast,* now paying attention to the aspects of subjectivation related to the encounter between the self and otherness.

2.2 Otherness in the literary text

As we have seen, in most of the stories in *Beauty and the Beast* there is an impactful and epiphanic moment when a character encounters another, with difference, an encounter that makes him reflect on himself and his own identity. In this sense, we believe that alterity will be the thematic and guiding thread of most of the plots in this work, which is why we allow ourselves to be led by this thread, towards new discoveries.

In the short story *Historia interrompida,* in which the character recounts her "affair" with a man she calls W... referring to this man's life, [in short] as a "pile of shards" (LISPECTOR, 1979, p. 15), the tone of the narrative is implicit, reiterated by the fragmented structure of the story (in "shards"), with complete passages and others such as "a lost hour", which she tries to "save or arrest". In this exercise in reminiscence, the narrator begins a long stitching together of threads and facts, aiming, above all, to give new meaning and re-significance to her own story, thus establishing her own identity.

Jane Pinheiro de Freitas, whose master's dissertation also studied the stories in *Beauty and the Beast*[5] , doesn't let this aspect of the construction of the self through the protagonist's imagination go unnoticed and states that: "It is in W.'s destructive tendency that the protagonist constructs herself, seeking her own identity through the other, she apprehends herself in the

[5]Jane Pinheiro de Freitas' research was carried out during her master's degree in the Postgraduate Program in Literary Theory at the University of São Paulo, under the supervision of Professor Ariovaldo Jose Vidal. The dissertation is, until now, the only research carried out in Brazil on the book *Beauty and the Beast,* by Clarice Lispector. We would also like to point out that, unlike the psychoanalytic bias observed in our work, Freitas' dissertation did not use psychoanalysis coro operate its interpretative reading.

ideas attributed to man, constructing her own identity through the characterization of W." (FREITAS, 2002, p.103).

In the narrative, the formation of this mosaic of "shards" resembles a chessboard, due to the repeated presence of the colors black and white - "So I sent for a cup of **coffee,** which he drank with a lot of **sugar and** greedily" (LISPECTOR, 1979, p.
16, emphasis added); "He was **dark** and sad [...] I was very **white** and happy, beside him." (LISPECTOR, 1979, p. 18, emphasis added); "I wanted to see if the **gray of** his words could blur my twenty-two years and the **clear** summer afternoon." (LISPECTOR, 1979, p.
17, emphasis added) - and the alternating movement of the characters. In this game, the narrative seems to alternate between processes of construction and deconstruction, in which "you destroy everything around you, but you can't destroy yourself and your desires (we have a body). Pure excuse." (LISPECTOR, 1979, p. 16). The narrator's words tell us that, in her search for identity, she follows clear and obscure paths, in a constant process of construction and deconstruction, guided mainly by the search for her desire.

Regina Pontieri (1999), writing an essay on alterity, states that the character turns her antagonist into a kind of "mirror in which to know herself, through similarity or antagonism" (PONTIERI, 1999, p. 104), which allows us to think that W... performs a specular function for the protagonist, similar to the one described by Freud in primary narcissism, on the road to self-identity.

The specular relationship between the characters is also evidenced by the narrative form. Let's see: **"He was dark and sad.** And he always **walked in the dark.** Oh, I certainly liked him. **Me, very white and cheerful,** next to him. Me, **in a flowery outfit,** cutting roses, **and him in dark, no, in white,** reading a book. Yes, we were quite a pair." (LISPECTOR, 1979, p. 18, emphasis added). In this excerpt, we perceive mirroring through antagonism, which brings us back to the game of mirrors mentioned by Moreira (2009), in which the other offers an image, a reflection, but is not really the subject.

Still in this sense, we remember a third character in the plot, the sister of the protagonist narrator and the only one with a proper name: Mira. Mira reminds us of "to look at", "to look at oneself" (in general, in the mirror, *mirror, an* English noun) and also allows us to conjecture that this name is yet another strategy by the author to draw the reader's attention to the specular function, mentioned earlier, in which the other offers an idealized image, with which the child initially identifies, but can later recognize himself as a unified being, separate from this other and also from this image.

Threatened by the constant possibility of destruction and finitude inherent in life, what remains and pulses strongly is the narrator's desire to find a way to save W..., to trap him. The protagonist narrator is seized by the desire to unite herself with the other, who, representing her opposite, would be the way to search for the self: "I wanted to find a formula that would give him to me. I wanted to find a formula that could save him. Yes, save him. And I liked that idea because it would justify the means I used to trap him" (LISPECTOR, 1979, p. 18).

The attempt to incorporate the male character takes us back to primary narcissism, when the infant experiences a fusion with the other, a fusion that prevents him from seeing otherness and something external to him. As we've seen, for a split to occur between the two subjects, castration anxiety is necessary, recognition of the difference, including sexual difference, which will enable the transition to secondary narcissism and libidinal investment in other objects.

This transition also seems to occur in the structure of the story, as the aforementioned passion undergoes a reversal in the narrative, as well as a change in other feelings and positions. There is a moment of tension in the narrative, in which the relationship between the two characters seems to swing between two poles, from love to hate, from admiration to dispute, and so a struggle begins between them. In the narrator's words: "Either I destroy him or he destroys me" (LISPECTOR, 1979, p. 16). This clash between the two characters, two forces, female vs. male, allows us to think about the conflict between the self and the narcissistic ideal offered by the privileged other, a conflict that makes us choose to separate from this other, to seek new paths and a less alienated ideal of the self.

The narrator thus seems to feel the need to break with this other, a break that was brought about by the abrupt death of the character W...:

> - Clarinha said he killed himself! He shot himself in the head... Is it true? It's a lie, isn't it?
> And suddenly the story broke. It didn't even have a smooth ending. It ended with the abruptness and lack of logic of a slap in the face (LISPECTOR, 1979, p. 21).

The death of W... signals the impossibility of incorporating him into it, as well as the impossibility of discovering or constructing a self and a static and definitive identity. The cutting of the narrative thread allows us to think about the difficult stitching of life, loose and fragmented by nature.

Despite such complexity, the protagonist narrator finds a way out for herself, a way of inscribing the self through the construction of her narrative. Perhaps this is where the author wants to alert us to aspects of life which, like the narrative, are more like a patchwork quilt, with countless gaps and loose threads, which each subject will have to artistically reconstruct.

In terms of an artistic reconfiguration, we see that many of the elements present in the plot of *An Interrupted Story - the* impact of the encounter with the other, attraction to its opposite, the desire for fusion, conflict between the self, identity and the other, alterity, the search for the inscription of the self through writing, among others - are also present in another short story, *Obsession,* albeit in a new configuration. This further highlights the talent of the writer Clarice Lispector, who represents the infinite possibility of saying, writing and, consequently, of being and living.

At this point, we will focus on analyzing how the elements discussed in the short story *Obsession* are configured.

As we saw in the first chapter, the story *Obsessaoë is* narrated by Cristina, who, after a lukewarm and happy childhood, followed by an equally lukewarm marriage to Jaime, falls ill and, alone, travels to Belo Horizonte in the hope of being cured. When she arrives in the city, she settles in a boarding house where she meets Daniel, a character she finds very attractive, mainly because of his antagonistic way of looking at life and his seductive dialogues, in which he reiterates the importance of desires in human life.

At the same time as she was strongly attracted to what Daniel represented, the narrator tried to avoid him, сото if she wanted to defend her amorphous life from anything that might disturb her comfort. But, as she herself says: "It was in vain. Daniel was the danger. And towards him I was walking". (LISPECTOR, 1979, p. 49).

Cristina takes it upon herself to describe Daniel's enigmatic personality and, although she has difficulty remembering his physiognomy (except for his smile), she attributes to him traits that could be reminiscent of a beast, with "long, curved fingers, those eyebrows that are far apart, dense" (LISPECTOR, 1979, p. 47), which further accentuates this aspect of danger and threat in the male character.

Freitas (2002) states that one of the ambiguities of the story is that Daniel is not exactly a danger, but rather the passage to that danger, which is more in Cristina than in Daniel himself. And so, over the course of the narrative, the "beautiful" narrator and protagonist reveals her "beast" side to the reader. Beginning to wonder about the cause of this transformation, the narrator says:

> Perhaps Daniel only acted as an instrument, perhaps my destiny was the one I followed, the destiny of those who are loose on the earth, of those who don't measure their actions by good or evil, perhaps even without him I would discover myself one day, perhaps even without him I would run away from Jaime and his land. What do I know? (LISPECTOR, 1979, p. 52).

In the midst of these doubts, it is important to describe this male character, who is initially constructed by the narrator in such a way as to reveal a man whose idea of life is linked to suffering, the desire for an eternal quest and a destructive personality. In Cristina's words: "I later got to know the real Daniel, the sick one, the one who only existed, albeit in perpetual clarity, within himself. When he turned to the world, already groping and faded, he found himself without support and, bitter, perplexed, he discovered that he only knew how to think." (LISPECTOR, 1979, p. 53). We can see from Cristina's descriptions that Daniel sought pleasure in an extremely narcissistic way, which excluded any kind of otherness, and ignored the dependence on the other, which was even necessary for the very process of identification.

However, Daniel will allow Cristina to approach him in one of the moments when he seems to need an opposite being, seeing in her a capacity to adapt to the world that he himself didn't possess. She identifies this and says: "Perhaps he would have allowed me to approach him at one of those moments when he needed the 'opposite force'". And yet: "And now I know, he tried so hard to crush me and humiliate me, because he envied me. He wanted to wake me up because he also wanted me to suffer, like a leper who secretly wants to pass on his leprosy to the saos." (LISPECTOR, 1979, p. 56).

The coming together of the two characters begins what Cristina calls her "transformation". At this point, she recounts the scenes she experienced with Daniel, and the reader can understand even more the role of the male character as an important instrument in the articulation of the plot.

In the short story *Obsessao,* Daniel can be seen as this instrument that will bring about a shock in the character Cristina, a transformation, in the words of the narrator: "Mad as hell, he repeated several times: he wanted to transform me, 'to blow into my body a little poison, the good and terrible poison...'" (LISPECTOR, 1979, p. 58). We notice in her allusion to poison an ambiguous aspect - good and terrible, in other words, the narrator seems to realize that entering the world of desire is also the awakening of the feminine and the human, and therefore, in her words, controversial: "Because I awoke simultaneously woman and human" (LISPECTOR, 1979, p. 52). In other words, life and suffering are intrinsically linked. This logic of interconnected life and suffering brings us back to Daniel's logic (and also that of the author Clarice), which the narrator grasps and says: "It sounds crazy. However, Daniel also had his logic. For him, suffering was contemplative, it was the only way to live intensely... And that, after all, was the only reason Daniel burned: to live. Only, his paths were strange" (LISPECTOR, 1979, p. 54). These are the paths the narrator will take, as she ends up succumbing to a new organization, just as oppressive as the previous one. This is because Cristina gives herself to Daniel, who acts as a substitute for Jaime's domesticated patriarchal power. In the words of Rosenbaum (1997): "Once again ready to be molded by the desire of the other, Cristina is now captured by Daniel's mental world and in it plays the role of victim with her tormentor, a projective screen of her lover's internal struggle." (p. 252).

At this point in the narrative, the dialogical spaces will be filled with Daniel's speeches, and Cristina's voice will no longer be heard, further emphasizing the narrator's submissiveness and passivity, as she no longer dares to express herself.

Captive of a still incomplete education, she has to return to "her previous life"; because of her mother's illness, she ends up returning to her home and to Jaime's side. However, she finds it difficult to readapt to the warm and dull environment, experiencing a sense of strangeness and anguish, which she describes as follows:

> I disguised my anguish and invented a pretext to withdraw for a few moments. In the bedroom, I would bite the tissue, stifling the cries of despair that threatened my throat. I fell into bed, my face sunk into the pillow, hoping that something would happen to save me. I began to hate them, all of them. And I wanted to abandon them, to run away from that feeling that developed with every minute, mixing a pity for them and for myself. As if together we were victims of the same irremediable hangover (LISPECTOR, 1979, p. 66).

This painful reunion is mainly due to the fact that her family members seem strange and incompatible with her "poisoned" conscience, in a process of constituting a self that finds no affinity with the family and increasingly distances itself from others and from itself. In this search to find herself, Cristina looks for the figure of Daniel: "After all, **what was I now, I felt, if not a reflection? If I abolished Daniel, I'd be a white mirror."** (LISPECTOR, 1979, p. 65, emphasis added). Here, we highlight Cristina's allusion to the mirror, which acquires importance in psychoanalytic theory, above all, a white mirror, reminiscent of the blank canvas. The importance of the mirror can also be seen in Clarice's writing:

> What is a mirror? It is the only invented material that is natural. Anyone who looks at a mirror, who can see it without seeing themselves, who understands that its depth consists in it being empty, who walks into its transparent shell without leaving a trace of their own image in it - that person has then understood its mystery as a thing. To do this, you have to surprise him when he's alone, when he's hanging in an empty room, without forgetting that the slightest needle in front of him could transform him into a simple image of a needle, so sensitive and mirror-like in its quality of light reflection, only an image and not a body. The body of the thing (LISPECTOR, 1973, p. 94).

In this excerpt, the author highlights the empty aspect of the mirror, which, despite being an invention, does not deny human nature, a nature that contains an emptiness, a fundamental lack. This is difficult for Cristina to see and feel, as she can't bear to face this emptiness and longs for the image obtained through Daniel, even if this image isn't what she really is.

The difficulty in facing o white mirror, that is, o emptiness, makes the narrator remain in "symbiosis with the other", as Rosenbaum (1997) puts it:

> Forged in the image and scmcllianca of a man, be he the representative of a deadly accommodation (coro Jaime), or the opposite extreme of the desperate restlessness of a spiral that abysses in on itself (coro Daniel), the woman prefers to lose her life in symbiosis with the other than to confront what she lacks. The "cure" would be a return to the white of the mirror, to emptiness, the constitutive hyalgia of a feminine that is always open and vulnerable (p. 257).

This symbiosis leads the protagonist to an imprisonment, regardless of the distance that separates her from Daniel. After all, the captivity she describes is first and foremost a mental imprisonment. Cristina, even in the absence of the other, inaugurates a substitute form of slavery:

> Often, thinking of him, in a slow transition, I saw myself serving him as a slave. Yes, I admitted, trembling and frightened: I, with a stable, conventional past, born into civilization, felt a painful pleasure in imagining myself at his feet, a slave... No, it wasn't love. It horrified me: it was degradation, degradation... (LISPECTOR, 1979, p. 68).

However, Rosenbaum (1997) warns that it is precisely this recognition of her imprisonment that, paradoxically, will allow the narrator to free herself, one of the greatest functions of Clarice's writing. After all, "although confusing, repetitive and incomplete, for Cristina (and her author) narration is, in the end, the only possibility of recovering her integrity and fidelity to herself". (ROSENBAUM, 1997, p. 259).

Although Daniel still posed a danger, the narrator believes that his presence was necessary for her desire for discovery and knowledge to survive; because of this, she decides to return to him, "like someone who nestles in the enemy's arms to be away from his arrows" (LISPECTOR, 1979, p. 68). Before returning to her beloved's side, she decides to leave a note for Jaime:

> With a sudden inspiration, I decided to leave Jaime a note, a note that would hurt Daniel! That o would leave him upset, crushed. And, just for the sake of showing Daniel that I was "strong", without any remorse, I deliberately wrote, trying to make myself distant and unattainable: "I'm leaving. I'm tired of living with you. If you can't understand me, at least trust me: I'm telling you that I'll be forgiven. If you were more intelligent, I'd tell you: don't judge me, don't forgive me, no one can do that. However, for your peace, forgive me." (LISPECTOR, 1979, p. 74).

Cristina thus seems to have taken on traces of Daniel's personality, discovering in herself a hostility previously reserved for her lover. At this point, there is a twist in the tale, driven by a dormant monstrosity - this "beast" hidden under the "beautiful". The relationship with Daniel takes on new traits, and the positions between them are slowly reversed - the dominator is placed in the position of a patient for whom she will be protection: "Gradually I took over his daily life, replaced him, like a nurse, in his movements. I took care of his books, his clothes, made his environment clearer." (LISPECTOR, 1979, p. 74). Far from awakening in her the longed-for vibration of existence, life with Daniel becomes lukewarm and silent, what the narrator calls an ideal death. The protagonist recounts: "I no longer listened to him as fervently, as exaltedly, as I used to. I had entered it. Nothing surprised me any more." (LISPECTOR, 1979, p. 75).

It was in this lukewarm and indifferent atmosphere that the climax of the story took place: Cristina's delay in returning home upset Daniel, displacing him from his position as sovereign. "For the first time I discovered that Daniel needed me! I had become necessary to the tyrant..." (LISPCETOR, 1979, p. 76). The incident generates *insight* in the narrator, while at the same time arousing disappointment, as all the power she had attributed to Daniel is exhausted. She says:

> Serviraja was my time as a slave. Perhaps I would continue to be one, without rebellion, until the end of my life. But I served a god... And Daniel had become weak, disenchanted. He needed me! I repeated it a thousand times afterwards, with the feeling that I had received a beautiful and enormous gift, too big for my brave men and for my desire. The strangest thing was that this impression was accompanied by another, absurdly new and strong one. I was free, I discovered at last... (LISPECTOR, 1979, p. 77).

Cristina seems to realize that Daniel's oppressive force has lost its meaning, having for a long time been the instrument that awakened her to the search for self-knowledge, but at that moment she sees that she hasn't completely molded herself to the other and that she needs to move on, looking for new paths: "What material am I made of where the elements and the basis of a thousand other lives intertwine but don't merge? I follow all the paths and none of them are mine yet. I've been molded into so many statues and I haven't stopped..." (LISPECTOR, 1979, p. 77).

On the walk alongside Daniel, feelings of intolerance and hatred begin to emerge, and the relationship between them takes on the nuances of a fight, with attacks and defenses: "We armed ourselves and were two forces" (LISPECTOR, 1979, p. 78). The new configuration of the relationship is also "invaded by habit" (LISPECTOR, 1979, p. 79), and the silence between the two characters emerges as an element of great significance, not as a weapon, but as a harbinger of an outcome: "There was a long pause, one of those that plunge you into awe. Everything stopped around us. [...] Like a new sigh, I came back to life. [...] - I'm leaving." (LISPECTOR, 1979, p. 81).

The sudden announcement of Cristina's departure creates a moment of truce and complicity between the two. The narrator and Daniel contemplate each other сото if they seek to reach a point of similarity, making converge, at the end of the narrative: love and hate, climax and anticlimax, aggression and friendship, "mysteries of what is human and at the limit unintelligible" (ROSENBAUM, 1997, p. 269).

The narrator says goodbye to Daniel and breaks away from the slavery to which she had become subject, experiencing the possibility of being her own subject. In the words of Rosenbaum (1997):

> Its exit, dramatized and then contained by the narrative, also represents an exit for language, which needs to self-engage in a painful autonomy. Freed from the tutelage of the other, without which, however, it cannot be constituted, subjectivity has had to prove itself and almost self-destruct in order to exist. Even so, it is in the confrontation with otherness that being can recognize itself (p. 271).

The narrator returns to Jaime, who accepts and respects her. However, she is not the same; she is now aware of her own loneliness and the continuing search for self-knowledge and for something that gives meaning to her own life. Cristina says: "As for me, I carry on. Alone now.

Forever alone." (LISPECTOR, 1979, p. 82).

The final sentences of the narrative are spoken in the present tense, bringing the narrator even closer to the reader and referring not only to the endless loneliness of being in search of a relationship, but also to the author's writing and solitary style. With regard to the act of writing, Clarice Lispector (apud BORELLI, 1981, p. 67) states that: "Writing is a solitary act, solitary in a different way from solitude". Although she writes alone, the writer seeks a dialogue with the other, the reader, and perhaps this is due to the different aspect of solitude.

Furthermore, with regard to the different types of loneliness, it is possible to think of the notion of the subject's helplessness, already mentioned in this dissertation, and realize that it is through the intermediary of the other and from a frightening and uncomfortable situation of helplessness that the subject is inserted into the field of language. For Rocha (2000), this condition of helplessness points to "the subject's dependence on the obscurity of the *Other's desire*. This inserts the subject into the *order of language* and, at the same time, translates helplessness into the experience of a *fundamental lack!"* (ROCHA, 2000, p. 113, emphasis added).

In this sense, each subject will look for ways to deal with the experience of this fundamental lack, and writing is one of them. Throughout Clarice's work, the questions of birth, origin, belonging and helplessness are part of the author's list of questions. Here, it's worth highlighting aspects of her biography, such as the fact that she was conceived in the hope that her mother would be cured. However, this was not possible, which makes her feel that she has failed in her mission. She describes:

> [...] I was prepared to be given birth in such a beautiful way. My mother was already ill, and it was widely believed that having a child cured a woman of a disease. So I was deliberately brought up: with love and confidence. Only I didn't cure my mother. And I still feel this burden of guilt to this day: I was made for a specific mission and I failed. As if they had counted on me in the trenches of a war and I had deserted. I know that my parents have forgiven me for having been born in vain and for having betrayed them in the great conspiracy. But I don't forgive myself. I wish that a miracle had simply happened: that I had been born and my mother healed. Then, yes: I would have belonged to my father and mother. I couldn't even trust anyone with this kind of loneliness of not belonging (LISPECTOR, 1999a, p. 111).

Faced with primordial helplessness, added to the experience of her birth as a failed mission, which attacks even the bond of belonging to her own parents, Clarice bears witness, in her writing, to the unspeakable anguish of such a situation. In her words: "The time to write is a reflection of a situation that is all my own. It's when I feel the greatest helplessness". (LISPECTOR, 1999b, p. 157).

Returning to the author's work, we realize that the "beast" aspects that began to emerge throughout the plot in the "beautiful" protagonist and narrator Cristina also refer us to another short story in the book, entitled *Beauty and the Beast or The Wound That's Too Big.*

The title of the short story opens up reflections on aspects that will run throughout the narrative, such as the encounter between opposites: beautiful and grotesque, male and female and other "oppositions" that lead to a "wound that is too big". In our view, this is a narcissistic wound experienced by the character Carla, narrated by a third person. Furthermore, the title suggests a parody of the children's fairy tale *Beauty and the Beast,* which also metaphorizes the union of the *beautiful and the* grotesque.

With regard to the narcissistic wound, we remember Freud's discussion of the narcissistic wound caused by psychoanalysis in humanity. In his essay *A Difficulty on the Road to Psychoanalysis* (1996f), Freud discusses his perception that psychoanalysis represents humanity's third narcissistic wound, preceded historically by the Copernican revolution in cosmology and the Darwinian revolution in biology. With Copernicus, the Earth was displaced from the center of the cosmos and placed in the secondary position of one of the many planets that revolve around the Sun; with Darwin, man lost his privileged place in nature, becoming a mere animal, derived from other species in biological evolution; with Freud, the last anchor of human pretension was removed, announcing that consciousness is no longer sovereign and that the self is not autonomous in this consciousness. What's more, psychic reality has shifted to the registers of the unconscious and the drive, which have come to regulate it. This further justifies the importance of deepening our understanding of these decentralizations, which are so significant to modern thought.

Returning to the story *A bela e a fera ou a ferida grande demais*, it's important to remember that it's narrated in the third person during the day of Carla de Souza e Santos, a lady from Rio who, on leaving the salon, comes across a beggar with a huge wound on his leg. The encounter between the two is striking, as it initially seems to be justified by the difference between the two characters, denounced by the allusion to their antagonistic thoughts: while the protagonist thinks "parties, parties, parties", the beggar thinks "food, food, food". In his analysis of the story, Freitas (2002) states that: "[...] the differences between the worlds of the two are accentuated, but metaphorically the two worlds come together. The woman compares the events of her life with that of the beggar, in a piano that goes from differences to similarities." (FREITAS, 2002, p. 39).

Initially, then, Carla's thoughts show the difference between them; the protagonist's mind is full of "silly" thoughts, сото: "[...] does this beggar know English? Has this beggar ever eaten caviar, drunk champagne?" (LISPECTOR, 1979, p. 138), until the moment when the thoughts are condensed into two words: "Social Justice." (LISPECTOR, 1979, p. 138). With "vision and understanding", Carla gradually unveils the life she leads, immersing herself in its intimacy and coming across great voids, which also leads her to a broader and more social view of their context, the context of the world. According to Freitas (2002):

> Along with the woman's questioning comes an awareness of the emptiness in which she lives, and the narrator shifts her to the position of victim as well, she, then, is сото other, and the product of a social system with its open wounds, and she who, with her assets, sustains the beggar's wound, but is "incapable" of sustaining herself in the face of that crisis. (FREITAS, 2002, p. 39).

The confrontation with this other lays bare what was previously supposed to be hidden, and otherness emerges as an uncomfortable force that disturbs the stability that existed before. Because of this, one of the protagonist's desires was to exterminate the source of that unease: "She had an unexpectedly murderous urge: to kill all the beggars in the world! Only so that, after the slaughter, she could enjoy her extraordinary well-being in peace". (LISPECTOR, 1979, p. 139)

That's because at the time of that encounter, Carla seemed to be enjoying a sense of well-being and good accommodation to the world in which she lived, and life seemed to be following its desirable rhythm, сото a well-functioning machine. But after the sight of the beggar, the impact seems to stop the movement, the action, making room for reflection. "Suddenly - suddenly everything stopped. The buses stopped, the people in the street stood still - only her heart beat, and for what?" (LISPECTOR, 1979, p. 138). In other words, the protagonist, who had been functioning as an important cog in the machine of life, seems to question her individuality, after all, "who was she?" (LISPECTOR, 1979, p. 142).

As we have seen throughout this chapter, the recognition of oneself is made possible after the recognition of otherness, in other words, the unveiling of oneself comes from the other, which, in Carla's case, comes through the image of this beggar, in whom she finds points of similarity and identification:

> - How come I never found out that I'm also a beggar? I've never asked for alms, but I beg for the love of my husband who has two mistresses, I beg for the love of God, that they find me beautiful, cheerful and acceptable, and my soul clothes are shabby... (LISPECTOR, 1979, p. 143)

Carla assumes that she is a beggar of emotions and feelings, a beggar of affection and of everything that ends up leading to him, and the resemblance between her and the beggar grows more and more. She reflected: "There are things that make us the same," she thought, desperately searching for another point of equality. Suddenly the answer came: "[...] they were equal because they had been born and they would both die. They were, therefore, brothers." (LISPECTOR, 1979, p. 144) The protagonist discovers points of equality and humanity between the two; however, the epiphanic moment of the story, in our opinion, of greatest revelation of the similarity between the two, refers to the capacity for language. A uniquely human capacity, shouted through the beggar's "toothless mouth" in the dialogue between him and Carla:

> Suddenly he asked the beggar:
> - Do you speak English?
> The man didn't even know what she had asked him. But, forced to answer because the woman had bought him with so much money, he took the evasive route:
> - Yes, I am. Why am I not talking to you right now? Why not? *Are* you deaf? Then I'll shout: FALO. (LISPECTOR, 1979, p. 142).

The beggar's cries seem to have echoed inside this woman, leading her to identify with this subject, mainly through language. Clarice purposely writes "FALO", in capital letters, in an attempt to shout in the reader's ears and emphasize the importance of language in the constitution of the subject. A theory reaffirmed by psychoanalysis, which also attributes other symbologies to the signifier "phallus"[6] .

Perhaps this is the greatest revelation of the encounter between Carla and the beggar: "Suddenly I knew: this beggar was made of the same material as her." (LISPECTOR, 1979, p. 144). The short story draws Lambern's attention to the possibility of revelation by other means, not only through the encounter with otherness, but also through the impact and revelation of the real[7] through art. This last aspect will be explored in greater depth in the next chapter.

Still on the subject of the encounter with otherness, we now turn to the short story *Gertrude asks for advice,* paying more attention to the meeting between the teenage Gertrude and the counselor who receives her letters, as already mentioned in the opening paraphrase of the story in the first chapter.

As we have seen, Gertrude seems to have grown up in an oppressive environment, in which thoughts must be repressed, giving way only to trivialities. "I don't like anything, I'm like the poets... Oh, not to think. Shame on you!" (LISPECTOR, 1979, p.26).

However, the protagonist's repressed thoughts seem to find space in the narrative, since the story is narrated in the third person by an observer who seems to hide in the character's consciousness, exposing her thoughts in particular. Thus, the restlessness that afflicts Gertrude, nicknamed Tuda, when she finds herself "mute" and unable to give voice to her desires, finds a solution in the voice of this narrator who seems to set her free. In the short story: "At other times, she was full of strength. Her gaze became as hard as sand, as rough as thorns. She felt

[6]The term "phallus" first appears in psychoanalytic theory in Freud and is later taken up by Lacan. According to Freud, the phallus is the organizing element of sexuality. This is because children's curiosity leads them to discover the anatomical difference between the sexes. However, the observation that a boy has something and a girl doesn't take the child beyond perceptual reality. The child will imaginatively construct their psychic reality, which presupposes that where they don't have something, something is missing. The notion of the lack of an object is therefore the result of the child's psychic elaboration of the anatomical difference between the sexes. The phallus is therefore the missing object. However, we can't confuse the term phallus with the penis, the male sexual organ, but rather with the representation that is constituted on the basis of this anatomical part. Lacan situates the phallus not merely as an organ of the body, nor as an imaginary object, nor even as a fantasy, but as a signifier, a symbolic operator that enables the subject to situate himself in the face of his desire: "Why speak of the phallus and not the penis? It's not a form or an image or a fantasy, but a signifier, the signifier of desire" (LACAN, 1998, p. 696). Therefore, the phallus is clarified by its function. The phallus allows the subject to represent himself in the face of what has no representation in the unconscious, that is, sexual difference, or sex.

[7]According to the *Dictionary of Psychoanalysis* (1998), the term "real" was used by Jacques Lacan, introduced in 1953 and taken simultaneously from the vocabulary of philosophy and the Freudian concept of psychic reality, to designate a phenomenal reality that is immanent to representation and impossible to symbolize. Used in the context of a topic, the concept of the real is inseparable from its other two components, the imaginary and the symbolic, and forms a structure with them.

she could. She had been made to 'liberate'. 'Liberate' was an immense word, full of mystery and pain." (LISPECTOR, 1979, p. 27).

It's interesting to note that сото Gertrudes, the Lambern narrator yearns for communication and correspondence, drawing the reader's attention to the importance of being understood and also of understanding the story Gertrudes experienced сото an adventure: "She lived in an atmosphere of fever and anxiety. An adventure. An adventure." (LISPECTOR, 1979, p. 28-29).

It seems important to "question" the reader, since the teenager is far from corresponding to the traditional heroine model in adventure narratives; on the contrary, she presents herself as the opposite of that heroine. In an exaggerated way, the narrator describes the teenager as if, despite her nickname Tuda, she felt like a "nothing", a being who has not yet been seen or understood by others, until the moment when she is called to the counselor's office[8] : "When she was called: they saw that she was something, an extraordinary, a misunderstood!" (LISPECTOR, 1979, p. 28). It should be emphasized that the invitation was not to go to a room, a consulting room, but "to the office", which brings us back, once again, to writing, in an allusion to the signifier, a verbal sign derived from "writing".

Unlike the traditional adventurous heroes' experiences of danger, conquests and fantastical feats, this teenager will take a risk in her encounter with the other and, consequently, with the possibility of recognizing herself. When Gertrude's eyes meet the doctor's vacant gaze and what it denounces, they catch the counselor's lack of affection. This is because the teenager, who until then hadn't gotten used to herself or the world, not knowing what to do with herself, bothered the woman, touching on her most intimate issues, reflecting her false attempts and "tricks" to mask her own unhappiness. The point of oppression seems to be common to both characters. However, they both feel uneasy about the impossibility of repressing their own desires and thoughts. The narrator is then mixed with the conscience of the counselor:

> He began to weaken and let himself be invaded by his own thoughts. He noticed it, got angry and transferred his irritation to Tuda: "So many people dying, so many 'homeless children', so many unsolvable problems (his problems) and that girl, with a family, a good bourgeois life, giving a damn". She vaguely observed that this ran counter to her individualist thesis: "Each person is a world, each person has their own key and that of others solves nothing; one only looks at the world of others out of distraction, out of interest, out of any other feeling that overshadows what is not vital; the 'evil of many' is consolation, but not a solution". (LISPECTOR, 1979, p. 32).

[8]It's important to note that Clarice Lispector also played the role of advisor at one point in her life.

From this excerpt of the narrative, we can scrutinize the counsellor's thoughts and thus see the impact that the encounter with the other also has on her. It seems difficult for the counselor to remain neutral; the teenager bothers her; she touches on her intimate issues, "her problems", making her look for general solutions that even escape her studies, values and what she often preaches as the truth. In this sense, we conjecture that the author Clarice Lispector perhaps wanted to emphasize the complexity of the encounter with the other and, consequently, perhaps ironize therapies, counseling, methods, after all, that use the discursive tool as the main working artifact.

With regard to psychoanalysis, however, we saw at the beginning of this chapter that the production of new meanings takes place in the paradoxical encounter between two absent selves, in a suspension of the control of the self, the opposite of what seems to happen between Gertrude and the counselor, when the latter begins to think about her own problems and judge the teenager's suffering on the basis of her own values.

The teenager seems to pick up on these thoughts unconsciously and realizes the discomfort she has caused the counsellor: "Suddenly, Tuda felt that the doctor didn't like her". (LISPECTOR, 1979, p. 32). At this point, the encounter between them takes on the tone of a duel and, in the intersubjective relationship, there is a point of contact, captured in the counselor's words to the girl:

> - Look, Tuda, **what I'd like to tell you** is that one day you'll have what you're so confused about right now. It's a kind of calm that comes from knowing yourself and others. But you can't rush this state. There are things you only learn when no one teaches you. And that's how it is with life. That's right. There's more beauty in discovering it alone, despite the suffering. The doctor felt suddenly tired. She had the impression that wrinkle number 3, from her nose to her lips, had sunk in. That girl was hurting her and she wanted to be alone again. - Look, I'm sure you'll still have a lot of happiness. Sensitive people are both unhappier and happier than others. But give it time! - Since he was easily vulgar, he reflected without bitterness - Go on living... [...] - Why did you say: "What would I like to tell you...? So it'*s* not the truth?" (LISPECTOR, 1979, p. 33-34, emphasis added).

In the doctor's words, Gertrude grasps the truth. This unconscious truth that apparently emerges is a mistake. We are reminded here of Freud's conceptualization of unconscious thought, thought marked by stumbling, by a truth that is always not all there is, always fractured, but which is nevertheless the only possible truth. A truth that the counsellor seems to recognize, while also acknowledging the perplexity of coming up against it:

> The girl was more perceptive than she had thought. No, it wasn't true. The doctor

> knew that you can spend your whole life looking for something behind the fog, and she also knew the perplexity that comes with knowing yourself and others. She knew that the beauty of life is small for those who look primarily for beauty in things (LISPECTOR, 1979, p. 34).

The contact with this fractured truth, and consequently with a more human dimension of the counselor, insofar as her "mistake" indicates a division, also placing her in the dimension of an incomplete being and not the holder of all truths, enables the teenager to finally find a correspondence for herself:

> Something had unfolded in her, her own personality that had taken hold with the certainty that there was a correspondence for her in the world... She was surprised: she could now talk about... "it" as something tangible, her dissatisfaction that she had hidden with shame and fear... Now... Someone had lightly touched the mysterious fogs she had been experiencing for some time and suddenly they had solidified, formed a block, existed. Until now, she had lacked anyone to recognize her, for her to recognize herself... Everything changed! How? I didn't know... (LISPECTOR, 1079, p. 36).

The transformation seems to take place even in the narrative form; initially, the narrator describes Gertrude and her emotions in an exaggerated way, sounding like an "annoying" person, and from the moment she identifies a lack in the other and comes into contact with her own lack, what initially seemed unbearable to her becomes palpable, indicating her own maturation, as well as that of the narrative itself.

The first moment of this transformation is also marked by a fusion - Gertrude and the counselor seem to become one, as we read in : "And suddenly Tuda felt that face entering deep into her soul. It wasn't the mouth or the eyes that brought that air... divine air" (LISPECTOR, 1979, p. 34). This epiphanic moment in the short story confirms Pontieri's (1999) observation that, in Clarice Lispector's fiction, it is possible to identify a "universal flesh" that all beings share, and that, for the writer, the experience of otherness shows that the other is not another me, but, on the contrary, the me is reduced to the condition of "other of the other".

This fusion is also accompanied by a subsequent separation, at the moment when Tuda sees himself as a "whole", an existing whole, unique and at the same time alone:

> His destiny had changed, it seemed to him. But coro? Oh, to not be able to think clearly and for **known words not to be able to express how she felt!** A little proud, a little dazzled, a little disappointed, she kept repeating: I'm going **to have another life, different from Amelia's, Mom's, Dad's...** She tried to envision a new future and could only see herself walking alone, her steps resolute, her eyes painful, walking, walking... Where to? (LISPECTOR, 1979, p. 37, emphasis added).

In this excerpt, we identify the adolescent's awareness of lack; a lack also marked in language, when she realizes that words cannot fully express what she feels. As we have seen, recognizing the lack makes it possible to separate from the primordial other, in a move towards secondary narcissism. Thus, the narrator describes Gertrude's thoughts: "to have another life, different from Amëlia, Mama, Papa". The character is thus able to follow another path, her own path, which is a source of pride and wonder and, at the same time, disappointment and anguish when she also realizes that she is a being in eternal helplessness.

The moment Gertrude feels this helplessness, the desire to return to that first state of fusion and satisfaction emerges:

> She felt suddenly depressed, without support. **She had been alone from one moment to the next... She wavered, disoriented. Where's Mom?** No, not Mom. Ah, to go back to the office, to look for the doctor's divine air, to ask her not to abandon her, because she was afraid, afraid! (LISPECTOR, 1979, p. 37, emphasis added).

Despite the fear of going it alone, the "hesitation" of wanting to regress to a previous situation of fusion with another, Gertrude chooses to recognize the lack, the fragmented truth, she chooses to inscribe herself. The narrator then describes the girl's thoughts: "A woman! The hidden power of this word. Because after all, **she thought, she... she existed! The** thought was accompanied by the sensation that she had a body of her own, a body that a man had looked at, a soul of her own, the soul that the doctor had touched." (LISPECTOR, 1979, p. 38).

From this excerpt, we realize that Gertrude's feeling that she had a body and a soul and, consequently, that she had an existence, did not emerge after she became aware that she was thinking, according to the Cartesian *cogito,* but, on the contrary, refers us to the new *cogito* proposed by Lacan in his *Writings.* "I think where I am not, therefore I am where I do not think" (LACAN, 1998, p. 521). Thinking is incompatible with the subject of the unconscious, being an operation of the self. Lacan takes the liberty of formulating what would be the Freudian *cogito*: *"Desidero, ergo sum"* (I desire, therefore I am), a desire that always points to something missing.

O desire points to lack, precisely because of the impossibility of its complete realization and satisfaction, which is what characterizes coтo the primordial aspect of the drive, which propelled Sigmund Freud to discover and elaborate the concept of the death drive, and which we will seek to understand in greater depth in the next chapter.

3 FROM REPRESENTATION TO PULSE

I'll tell you a secret: life is deadly. (LISPECTOR, 1980, p. 77)

So far, we have followed the directions pointed out by Birman (2003) about the two movements of de-centering of the idea of the subject operated by psychoanalysis, that is, in the first movement, with the discovery of the unconscious and the consequent Freudian formulations around a psychic reality, in which fantasy and affections produce concrete values over subjectivity, the self and consciousness lose their prevalent value for animic life. In the second movement, also in the direction of a deconstruction of the subject built on reason and consciousness, Freudian theorizing displaced this subject from the self to the other, placing it outside of itself. Thus, in this chapter, we come to the last and third movement, from representation to drive.

According to Birman (2003), the two initial decenterings had representation on the agenda, and it is precisely representation that will undergo a decentering in the third movement. This means that, from the moment Freud introduces the concept of the death drive, a drive without representation, a pure force in movement, producing rupture and dispersion, the axis of representation, until then capable of integrating experience with oneself and with others, will no longer be possible. The existence of a field that escapes theorization thus places a limit on representation.

In order to better understand this movement, it is necessary to delve into Freud's discovery of the death drive, as well as his formulations about a drive-based self.

3.1 O pulsional self

The term pulse, first found in Freud's work in the edition of *Three Essays on the Theory of Sexuality* (1996b), is defined as the psychic representative of constant stimuli from an endogenous source, and is therefore a limiting concept between the psyche and the somatic.

In this text, Freud introduces the partial pulses linked to specific erogenous zones, the sum of which would constitute infantile sexuality. Although they are linked to infantile sexuality, these erogenous zones are active throughout life, functioning in the form of preliminary pleasures and perversions in adulthood, or even under the fate of repression. E

The plasticity of the drive is also evident, in other words, Freud states that the drive is capable of adapting to a multitude of objects, so that its object and personality are the most variable aspects of the drive.

Later, Freud enunciated his first drive dualism, introducing the concept of the drive of the self. As we saw in the previous chapter, in the first Freudian topic, the psychic conflict was between the sexual drive, in the service of sexuality, and the drive of the self, in the service of the individual's conservation. In the text *Formulagoes sobre os dois principios do funcionamento mental* (1996b), the father of psychoanalysis goes into more detail about this psychic conflict, subjecting the sexual drive to the dominance of the pleasure principle and the drive of the self to the dominance of the reality principle.

In 1914, with the introduction of narcissism and the discovery of libidinal investment in the self and, therefore, of a self that is also the object of sexual libido, Freud would subvert the first drive dualism and present a second: libido of the self (sexual drive invested in the self) and object libido (sexual drive invested in objects).

Based on his clinical observations, Freud saw the need and importance of deepening his studies on the concept of the drive and, a year later, he rescued such theorizing in his text *Instincts and their vicissitudes* (1996e). In this text, he rectified his initial concept and, at the same time, foreshadowed the propositions he would develop in *Beyond the Pleasure Principle* (1996g), when he began to oppose life and death impulses.

In *Instincts and Their Vicissitudes* (1996e), Freud reintroduces the elements about the functioning of the drive coтo: source *[Quelle]* (somatic process that occurs in an organ or part of the body, but, in terms of the mental pathway, we only get to know it through the purposes of the drive); Fmality *[Ziel]* (satisfaction that can only be achieved through the elimination of the state of stimulation, achieved through a direct path or through the combination of various closer or intermediate goals that combine and interchange with each other in order to reach the ultimate fmality); and object *[Objekt]* (it is through an object that the drive is able to achieve its fmality). He adds one more element, pressure *[Drang], which is* characterized by being a constant pressure and is the very essence of the pulse. It is its driving factor, its amount of force configured as a demand for work from the psyche. For Freud, every drive is active, and one can only speak of drive passivity when referring to formality.

As such, the drive is fundamentally a constant force, permanently demanding work on the psyche, in a movement to discharge its excitability, since the organism has no regulators of this excitability. In this essay, Freud also introduces the novelty of the transformation from a quantitative to a qualitative dimension and, consequently, the importance of otherness in this process. This is because, since the pulse is a force that inhabits the border between the psychic and the somatic, it is necessary to submit this energetic *quantum* to the process of symbolization in order to achieve a qualitative register and thus make it possible to inscribe the force. Moreira (2009) describes this process:

> In order for the drive, coro force, to be transformed into a drive circuit, in which this energy is articulated with the dimension of the other-object, and to be inscribed in the field of satisfaction, it is necessary to do the work of offering possibilities for satisfaction. This work is carried out by the other, who offers the drive a variety of objects for its satisfaction (MOREIRA, 2009, p. 244).

This makes us understand that the interference of the other is fundamental in the drive field for the passage from the biological to the psychic, enabling the reception and transformation of such excitability.

As there are no devices in the psyche to regulate such excitability, nor the capacity to capture it, the lack of another capable of receiving such a discharge would imply the death of such an organism, since the total elimination of the organism's excitability would imply this. This is where we see a new Freudian thermodynamic concept, which alludes to the need to accommodate and transform this constant force, so that this excitability is not simply eliminated, as this would imply the death of the organism itself.

Unlike the vitalist assumptions of the first topic, in which the organism was made up of a homeostatic system of self-regulation, whose vital imperative was the maintenance of life, in the second topic, Sigmund Freud enunciates the incapacity of the human organism to regulate itself, and death is now the original movement of this organism.

In view of this, Freud deepened his studies and presented in *Beyond the Principle of Pleasure* (1996g) a new drive dualism: the opposition between the life drive and the death drive.

In the words of Birman (2003):

> The movement towards absolute discharge would now be carried out by the death drive, heir to the concept of the drive, which would be opposed to the life drive, operated by the other. Human biological life would now be strictly dependent on the erotic investment of the other, who would provide the regulation that the organism does not have for itself. This implies that the order of life, as far as the human organism is concerned, would strictly depend on an organization promoted by the other. In this way, human life would not be something of nature, but also of artifice and construction, always provided by the other. (p. 22).

In this sense, the organism aspires to absolute stillness, the principle of nirvana, making the principle of reality and the agency of the other responsible for the construction of the drive circuit and the experience of satisfaction. This gives life aspects of construction, transformation and the creation of artifices against an organism primarily focused on death.

Faced with the restlessness of the drive, there will be countless destinations for the drive: attitudes, movements, different Iagos will form between the drive and its objects and representatives, and this is the path of the constitution of the subject. This means that, from this new Freudian perspective, not only does life take on aspects of construction, but the very constitution of identity undergoes re-evaluation, so that the existence of a drive without representation can lead the subject to direct their drive towards the creation of their singularity, the search for new destinies and new possibilities of subjectivation. Although it is not of the order of language, the death drive encourages and forces the subject to create new possibilities of expression.

In the essay *The instincts and their vicissitudes* (1996e), Freud also discusses the possible destinations for the drive: repression, reversal into its opposite, return to the self or sublimation. This is extremely important for understanding our work, insofar as it enables creation under the demands of the unnameable and, in this sense, reaches artistic creation, our object of study.

3.2 Sublimation, the creationist powerhouse

The concept of sublimation appears in a fragmented and disseminated form throughout Freud's work and, although there is no essay dedicated exclusively to it, it is considered to be of fundamental importance for psychoanalysis. Considering its importance also for the discussion of our work, we will try to trace these fragments, paying particular attention to their articulation with the concept of pulse, which opens up the possibility of creation.

It was in the case of Dora[9] , published in 1905, that sublimation was introduced by Freud, who used the term in his correspondence with Fliess[10] . Its first appearance brings together ideas underlying its conceptualization, which will remain until the end of the work:

[9]The Dora case refers to Sigmund Freud's first major treatment of the patient Ida Bauer. The story of Dora, as the psychoanalyst named it, was written in December 1900 and January 1901 and published four years later, taking place between the publication of *The Interpretation of Dreams* and *Three Essays on the Theory of Sexuality*. Over the years, the text has acquired a particular status, being one of the most talked about clinical documents since its publication. This is because it was mainly through the reporting of this case that Freud sought to give validity to his theses on hysterical neurosis and to expose the nature of psychoanalytic treatment, already based on dream interpretation and free association, and no longer on the method of catharsis and hypnosis.

[10] Wilhelm Fliess was a German doctor, close friend of Freud and theorist of bisexuality. According to the *Dictionary of Psychoanalysis* (1998), it was in October 1887, during a stay in Vienna, that Fliess met Sigmund Freud. The two doctors were interested in sexuality, looking to medicine and science for ways to build a new theory of human psychic life. Their friendship was passionate and was accompanied by a great deal of correspondence, of which unfortunately only the part written by Freud is known. They contain numerous discussions and psychoanalytic hypotheses, as well as a multitude of details about the daily and sexual life of the father of psychoanalysis. Their correspondence ended in September 1902 after a violent break in their friendship.

sublimation is a defense mechanism against impulses; it deforms and modifies unpleasant content; it implies a change of goal from sexual impulses towards socially elevated goals; it provides the driving force for many cultural achievements.

The theses announced in the Dora case are developed in the aforementioned *Three Essays on the Theory of Sexuality* (1996b), in which Freud situates the drives that will be the target of sublimation in sexual development, circumscribing, for the first time, the concept of sublimation. It's important to note that in that essay, sublimation becomes an operation of deviation from the primary goal of the sexual drive - the original goal - towards a non-sexual target. Let's see:

> The progressive concealment of the body brought about by civilization keeps sexual curiosity aroused, which aspires to complete the sexual object through the recreation of the hidden parts, but which can be diverted ("sublimated") into art, if it is possible to remove interest from the genitals and turn it towards the shape of the body as a whole (FREUD, 1996b, p. 148).

This passage is quite interesting, mainly because it highlights two aspects: the first refers to the notion of deviation como overtaking, so that in this deviation, something of the sexual would not be lost in its journey to the non-sexual - it would alёт, in some way, continue with it and deviate from it; the second aspect refers to the association of the mechanism of sublimation with artistic activity.

The term deviation marks an important difference between the mechanism of sublimation and repression: in the former, the pulse is diverted from its target, leaves the reference to direct sexual satisfaction and deals with it in the dimension of the impossible, whereas in repression, the subject remains attached to the sexual, which is the point of reference for him, at the level of the forbidden. As such, sublimation is considered to be an outlet for impulses without involving repression. This brings us back to the concept of sublimation from the point of view of chemistry, in which it is considered to be the direct passage from the solid to the gaseous state, without passing through the liquid state. In other words, in sublimation, the drive retains its sexual content, modifying its purpose, which shifts from the sexual to the social, without necessarily involving the mechanism of repression.

With regard to the link between sublimation and artistic activity, in 1908, in the text *Creative Writers and Daydreams,* Freud discusses the dimension of creation that operates both in children's activities and in sublimatory activities, the latter being related to literary creation. When addressing the relationship between literary creation and children's play, Freud asks himself: "Could we not say that in playing every child behaves like a creative writer, because he creates a world of his own, or rather readjusts the elements of his world in a way that pleases him?" (FREUD, 1996c, p. 135). As Valle (2006) points out, "this text is timely in that it sets out Freud's conception of sublimation as the creation of new objects and spaces to meet sexual demands, both on the part of the creative writer and on the part of the reader who comes into contact with the work". (p. 53).

Freud would later return to the relationship between artistic creation and sublimation in other texts - such as the article on Leonardo da Vinci, in which he dealt with sublimation as an erotic movement that has its roots in childhood. However, we won't dwell on the analysis of these texts, but only pay attention to the traces they leave behind and enable us to think of sublimation as a fundamentally creative movement.

The sublimatory aspect, in terms of the creation of new possibilities, is concretized mainly in 1930, in *The Malaise of Civilization* (FREUD, 1996h). In this work, Freud further discusses the aspect of civilization that rests on the coercion of sexual impulses and the ways in which human beings have found to deal with this aspect. In this text, sublimatory activity appears to be a defense technique against suffering, because it promotes libidinal displacement and produces types of satisfaction accepted by the outside world. In his words:

> Another technique for warding off suffering lies in using the displacements of libido that our mental apparatus makes possible and through which its function gains so much flexibility. The task here consists of reorienting the drive's objectives in such a way as to avoid frustration from the external world. To do this, it relies on the sublimation of the impulses. Maximum satisfaction is achieved when the production of pleasure is sufficiently intensified from the sources of psychic and intellectual work. When this happens, fate can do little against us. Satisfaction of this kind, for example, the joy of the artist in creating, in embodying his fantasies, or that of the scientist in solving problems or discovering truths, has a special quality that we will undoubtedly one day be able to characterize in metapsychological terms. [...] The weakness of this method is that it is not generally applicable, since it is only accessible to a few people. It presupposes the possession of special skills and dispositions which, for any practical purpose, are far from common. And even for the few who do possess them, the method does not provide protection against suffering. It doesn't create impenetrable armor against the onslaughts of fate and usually fails when the source of suffering is the person's own body (FREUD, 1996h, p. 87).

In this passage, we highlight Freud's mention of the suffering inherent in human life and the inability of the sublimatory mechanism to totally annihilate it. In this sense, we understand that sublimation brings with it the fundamental aspect of the drive: the impossibility of its full satisfaction. Thus, suffering and lack are present, making its connection with sublimation vivid. It is precisely from this lack, this emptiness and this non-sense that the subject will be led to create new investments, new encounters, new meanings.

Still in the text *The Evil State of Civilization,* Freud situates sublimation as a ethical issue, since, in analysing the impossibility of full satisfaction of the drive and, consequently, the unfeasibility of happiness in the full sense, he begins to reflect on the manoeuvres possible for the subject in order to achieve something less uncomfortable for himself. He says:

> The program of becoming happy, which the pleasure principle imposes on us, cannot be achieved; however, we must not - indeed we cannot - abandon our efforts to get closer to achievement, one way or another. Very different paths can be taken in this direction, and we can prioritize either the positive aspect of the goal, obtaining pleasure, or the negative aspect, avoiding displeasure. Neither of these paths leads to everything we want. Happiness, in the limited sense in which we recognize it as possible, is a problem of the economy of the individual's libido. **There is no golden rule that applies to everyone: every man has to discover for himself in what specific way he can be saved.** All sorts of different factors will operate to direct his choice. It's a question of how much real satisfaction he can expect to derive from the external world, how far he is driven to become independent of it, and, finally, how much power he feels at his disposal to alter the world in order to adapt it to his desires. In this, his psychic constitution will play a decisive role, independent of external circumstances (FREUD, 1996h, p. 90-91, emphasis added).

Freud is telling us about a singular aspect of subjective inscription, a unique way found by each subject to modify their relationship with suffering, in the sense that sublimation has the particularity of transforming the destinies of the drive. Lacan re-reads Freud's mechanism of sublimation and, by articulating it with the negation of the death drive, elaborates what he calls "creationist sublimation". (LACAN, 1988, p.
259-261). For him, there is an important point of connection between the death drive (a deadly movement that he called jouissance), fantasy and sublimation, insofar as, in order to confront this annihilating tendency, unconscious fantasy will clothe nothingness, giving it contours, creating something out of it. In other words, creationist sublimation would be something that, in the face of imminent destruction, renews itself and makes the terrifying abyss of emptiness act as a source of constant creation for the originally helpless life, thus situating it as a movement inherent to the subject, a structural movement of renewed attempts to construct new meanings and new possibilities of some comfort and place for their desires.

In this sense, art repeats the model of this creationist power, in that it is also a conception from nothing, a creation that works with the void, unlike religion and science, which Freud also mentions in *The Malaise of Civilization.* According to the father of psychoanalysis, art differs from religion in that religion tries to fill the void, and desire is often seen as a sin, with its redemption in prayers and absolutions. The meaninglessness of death is filled by the promise of eternal life. Science, on the other hand, rejects emptiness and constantly seeks ways to appease it. It presents itself as complete knowledge and keeps the individual subordinate to it. For Lacan, art recognizes the void and makes it the cause of creation, something that can be produced in its surroundings.

Lacan's elaboration reminds us that writing is a creative experience, and here we find Clarice Lispector's writing, in its transformative and revealing yearning for anguish and desire. Ana Maria Lima do Valle discusses the relationship between Clarice's writing and the creationist sublimation elaborated by Lacan, in her dissertation entitled *Clarice Lispector's Writing in the Transmission of the Real.* In relation to Clarice's writing, she says:

> Writing that often soars in intense contradiction. Moments of extreme search for death, for rapid and absolute destruction, at others of luminous renewed joy. Sunny moments where life pulses, hope lifts its gaze to the horizon and joy is truly possible. Despite the undeniable pain (VALLE, 2006, p. 96).

We've observed that the contradictory and heightened movement between the deadly and vital tendencies in Clarice's writing also brings us back to the movement of the subject in the face of drive demands, in the face of emptiness and constituent helplessness. In our analysis of the short stories in *Beauty and the Beast,* we will now pay attention not only to the movements between the self and otherness, but also to the alternating movements of the subject's life drive and death drive and their representations throughout the plot - alternating movements, but fundamental to enabling psychic organization and, consequently, the organization of the self and of the literary text.

We will then make a move similar to the third Freudian de-centering, starting from the representation of the text, to get in touch with pulsational aspects and even with the impossibility of representation, in the certainty that we will be treading on rough terrain, to which literature takes us.

3.3 Death and life in Clarice Lispector's short stories

As we have seen, Clarice Lispector's writing includes contradictory aspects: it ranges from joy to sadness, from security to insecurity, from life to death, making this range of emotions and sensations accessible to the reader. Rosembaum (1997) also points out that Clarice's writing frustrates the desire for consolation, constantly bringing the reader back to the unease of uncertainty, dissociated fragments and loss of reference.

Continuing our analysis of the short stories, now paying attention to the vital and deadly aspects of this writing, we bring up for discussion the short story *One Day Less,* also found in *Beauty and the Beast.*

The short story entitled *One Day Less* narrates, in mirrored first and third person, the tedious day of a 30-year-old woman, whose name is Margarida das Flores, but who has been nicknamed Margarida Flores de Enterro since childhood. The noun burial, as well as the reiteration of the word death and, above all, the narrator's initial reverie, sensitize us to the morbidity of the character's life, as well as anticipating the end of the story when the protagonist is supposed to have committed suicide. The story opens with the narrator's first-person reflection on the existence of death: "I suspect that death is coming. Death? [...] Will the long days ever end? [...] So I daydream calmly, quietly. Is death a bluff? A trick of life? Is it persecution? [...] And so it is." (LISPECTOR, 1979, p. 119).

The days seem to tire this character, who doesn't work (since her parents' pension provides for her few needs), but also has no leisure time or any kind of apparent personal fulfillment. The narrative has diary-like aspects, recounting the stages of this woman's day: waking up, eating, reading, watching TV, smoking, eating, sleeping, all of them narrated in an automatic and impersonal tone. Aside from the daily activities that fill her day, Margarida is driven by memories of the past and of dead people, witnessing nothing new in her own existence.

The character who "by mere chance was born" (LISPECTOR, 1979, p. 120), who is extremely lonely, searches for references, for something else to guide her and to tidy herself up, in the same way that she tidies her panties and underwear:

> [...] she was exactly the type to sort out drawers of knickers and underwear, and she felt good about the delicate task. And if she were married, her husband would have the row of ties in perfect order, according to color gradation, or according to... According to anything. Because there's always something to be guided by. When she was herself, she was guided by the fact that she wasn't married, that she'd had the same maid since birth, that she was a woman in her thirties, with little lipstick, pale clothes... and what else? (LISPECTOR, 1979, p. 122).

It's interesting that the words "guiar" and "arrumar" are close to each other, both referring to a path, a direction, which leads us to think of the need for something to guide oneself, not just in everyday tasks, but mainly to take a direction on one's path, perhaps the desire that drives the subject in their quests.

In this case, if Marguerite, in the absence of new events, is moved by past things, feeling that she still has no references, she is in a state of living death, as if she had no existence. One of the aspects that illustrates this is that стелca is the most odorless of creatures and, looking for a sign of existence, compulsively passes talcum powder around: "After the bath and the thoughts, talcum powder, talcum powder, lots of talcum powder. And how many deodorants: I doubted that anyone in Rio de Janeiro smelled less than her. Perhaps she was the most odorless of creatures." (LISPECTOR, 1979, p. 122). The absence of this bodily sense and the lack of traits that define her personality signal a difficulty in affirming her own identity, also reaffirmed by the difficulty the character has in looking at herself in the mirror: "She rarely saw herself in the mirror, as if she already knew too much" (LISPECTOR, 1979, p. 121). However, this character seems to lack an other who recognizes her and, consequently, enables her own self-knowledge.

Loneliness is a striking theme in the story, as the character finds herself absolutely alone: her parents are dead and her maid - the only person with whom she has a strong emotional bond - has spent a month's vacation visiting her son. In an attempt to connect with someone, the character longs for a phone call. She daydreams that a man might call and invite her for afternoon tea. But her thoughts are interrupted by a sense of inadequacy for her time, since an invitation for a drink would be more likely, not a cup of tea.

Immersed in the routine activities of her day, Margarida is surprised by the ringing of the telephone:

> IT HAPPENED! I swear, she **said, I** swear I heard the phone ring. She spat on the towel after eating her third piece of toast and, so as not to make it look like she was being hasty or needy, she let it ring four times, and each time it was a sharp pain in the heart because they might hang up thinking there was no one home! At this terrifying thought, she suddenly rushed to that same fourth call and managed to say in a very negligent voice:
> - Aid... (LISPECTOR, 1979, p. 125, emphasis added).

In this excerpt, we notice a muffled self, as the protagonist seems to say to herself that the phone had rung. Contrary to what she had dreamed, on the other end was not a male voice, but a female voice "who must have been over eighty, judging by her hoarse drawl" (LISPECTOR, 1979, p. 125), also lonely, looking for someone called Flavia to play a game of cards with. When she informs the lady, named Constanta, that there is no one with that name on the number dialed, the two characters start an argument, right at the moment of asking about Margarida's name:

> - Stop being rude, you little bitch! By the way, what's your name?
> - Margarida Flores do Jardim.
> - Why? Are there flowers in the garden?
> - Ah, ah, ah, you're in a good mood! No, there are no flowers in the garden, but my name is flowery.
> - Is that any good?
>
> Silence.

> - Is there any point, or is there no point?
> - And I don't know how to answer because I've never thought about it before. I only know how to answer things I've thought (LISPECTOR, 1979, p. 126).

Madame Constanta's question accentuates Margarida's loneliness and unhappiness even more, as well as her contempt for herself, since "she had never stopped to think about whether or not she was happy." (LISPECTOR, 1979, p. 128). The confrontation with this woman places the protagonist in front of a mirror where she gets to know herself.

However, this "mirror" and Margarida's thoughts seem to have shown her painful aspects of her existence, leading her to "naively" take all the insomnia pills that had belonged to her mother. It's interesting that the narrator alludes to this act of the protagonist with extreme subtlety, since, in this case, the protagonist's act of suicide takes on ambiguous overtones and her death also represents a liberation for her, her "debut" is a new birth:

> He didn't notice the slightest intrusion in himself. But no one in the world will ever know. And now, forever, you won't be able to tell if it was due to an imbalance or finally a great balance: glass after glass, you swallowed all the pills in the three large glasses. But in the second glass he thought for the first time in his life: "Me". And it wasn't just a rehearsal: it was actually a premiere. She was finally making her debut (LISPECTOR, 1979, p. 129).

Margarida seems to be making her debut as a subject, insofar as she takes the step of asserting a desire rooted in this death drive. She then dies in the same bed where she was born, making her reverie real, ending the pursuit of death and bringing an end to endless days. "It was one day less" (LISPECTOR, 1979, p. 130).

From the excerpt above, we can also think of the metamorphosis of this character, who used to be "She", but finally emerges as an "I", and experiences her debut as a narrator. A narrator who had to "kill" this "she" in order to emerge as an "I".

Freitas (2002), in his research on the presence of an anticipation of important aspects of Clarice's writing in her first short stories, points out that the fact that Margarida fell on her parents' bed, dying in the same place where she was born, refers to the question of circularity, which is very present in Clarice's work. In other words, in the short story analyzed, it is clear that Lispector used the strategy of figuratively tying the two ends of existence together: life and death. This movement will also recur in her future writing, for example, in the form of the book *A Breath of Life. Pulsations.* Let's remember: "I've read this book to the end and I'm adding some news in this regard. It means that the end, which shouldn't be read before, splices itself in a circle with the beginning, a snake that swallows its own tail." (LISPECTOR, 1978, p. 20). Similarly, the questioning of death, seen at the beginning of the short story *Um dia a menos,* also anticipates this aspect that will emerge at the end of the text.

The short story *Um dia a menos* also presents other recurring aspects of Clarice's work; here we highlight some similarities with the novel *A hora da estrela,* starting with the year the book was published and written - 1977. As it was the last novel the writer published during her lifetime, months before her death, *The Hour of the Star* arouses interest and curiosity, both because it seems to be Clarice Lispector's literary testament and because it demands of its reader a kind of continuous reminiscence of the novels that preceded it, since the themes and situations experienced by the characters reverberate in the novel in question.

We can see that in both plots - the short story *Menos um dia* and the novel *A hora da estrela* - there is a repeated problematic of identity: both Margarida and MacaЬёa (the protagonist of *A hora da estrela)* explore a search, albeit unconscious, for a unified self-image. In the case of MacaЬёa, this search seems to take place through the narrator Rodrigo S. M. and his continued efforts to construct this character.

Still in the context of the search for identity, we identified a sense of strangeness in relation to their own names in both characters. This strangeness is aroused mainly after the encounter with otherness. In the short story, we see that when Constanta asks her if her life has flowers in it, Margarida is faced with doubt and, consequently, with the awareness of an existence that is not very flowery, not very felt or experienced. Macabda[11] , when she meets Olimpio, her boyfriend, sees that he reacts with astonishment because he doesn't understand her name, which goes hand in hand with the lack of knowledge of her own being, identified in one of her lines: "I don't know what's inside my name." (LISPECTOR, 1998a, p. 56). This lack of knowledge about the meaning of their own name, as well as their own being, is the cause of anguish for both characters.

If aт the name, we also conceive of language coтo a source of revelation granted to the individual, all it takes is for it to be captured, we touch on the heart of the problem of MacaЬёa and Margarida: both are deprived of the power of communication because they are constructed by another, by the narrator. In the case of MacaЬёa, this narrator is identified as Rodrigo S. M. However, this power of communication will be rescued at the end of the narratives, in which there will be the death of the "she" for the emergence (debut/star) of an "I".

After identifying so many similarities between the narrative of the short story *One Day Less* and The *Hour of the Star,* we remember Vilma Areas, who, in her book *Clarice Lispector com a ponta dos dedos* (2005), points out that Clarice's most significant texts, and here we can

"O поте Maccabaeus" refers to the biblical Maccabees and, above all, to Judas Maccabaeus, who was a Jewish leader who organized an army to resist the Greek occupation of Jerusalem. Because of this, the Maccabees were recognized as fearless creatures in the face of the world.

include *The Hour of the Star,* came in a slow gestation through varied narratives of different weights over time, coто the work of someone who had been practicing scales on the piano. We believe that the tales in *Beauty and the Beast* are also constituents of this Claricean melody - their texts vary in tone, but do not lose their importance in the constitution of the music as a whole.

Listening carefully to Clarice's music and, consequently, perceiving its different tones, has sharpened the apprehension of deadly and vital signifiers. We endorse this statement by returning to Freudian theorizing about the pulses of life and death, when he affirms the mixture between them and the variety of ways in which these pulses manifest themselves, with the death pulse often manifesting itself silently.

We understand the work of art to be a space for the management of these pulses - the act of writing, despite being permeated by the death drive, is an activity of producing meaning, of connection - making it possible to order the circuits of the drive in the register of symbolization and its circulation coто the aesthetic object and pleasure. It's as if he transformed death into life. The word itself is a vital impulse, as Clarice herself says: "I write as if to save someone's life. Probably my own life". (LISPECTOR, 1978, p.ll).

This is one of the most important aspects of artistic activity: at the same time as things are unreachable, art establishes a place where not only the intensity and excess of the drive can be present, but also the possibility, through artistic creation, of structuring reality in a personal and stylized way, constituting possible destinations for the drive forms and inscribing the drive in the register of symbolization. In this sense, the act of artistic creation is very similar to the creation of the subject and the psychic effort they have to make in order to organize their drives in a process of constructing their own identity.

Reading and analyzing the tales of *Beauty and the Beast* allowed us to identify countless possible destinations for these drive forms in different registers of symbolization and narrative forms. In addition, we followed the characters' struggle to deal with their own "chaos" of drive. Let's remember.

In the first story, *Historia interrompida,* the narrator, through writing, tries to weave aspects of her story and understand the sudden death of W.... In the process, she describes her desires, including the desire to arrest W..., which are suddenly interrupted by the man's death. Despite this emptiness, caused by the inevitability of death, its destructive aspect and its rupture, she searches for symbolization, for the possibility of connection and, for this reason, she bets on the act of writing. As she describes:

> And I only wrote "this" to see if I could find an answer to the questions that torture me from time to time, disturbing my peace: what was the meaning of W...'s passage through the world? what was the meaning of my pain? what is the thread that these facts have to... "Eternity. Life. World. God." (LISPECTOR, 1979, p. 21).

In the second story, *Gertrude asks for advice.* We saw that the adolescent Gertrude's desire to understand the world and herself was not paralyzed by her desire to die or by life's misunderstandings, as she wrote in her correspondence to the doctor: "I've already decided to commit suicide, but I don't want to anymore. Can you help me? Gertrudes." (LISPECTOR, 1979, p. 25). The search for contact with this doctor is also a search for an encounter with the other, for a connection, which also represents a pulse of life.

This ambiguity can be seen above all in the third story, *Obsession,* in which we learn about the love-hate relationship between Daniel and Cristina, the encounters and disagreements they experience and the complexity involved in this bond. This complexity and depth merited a warning to the reader from the narrator Cristina: "You know how much is enough to transform the atmosphere in which two people live. A small gesture, a smile hooks onto one of the feelings that lie tangled at the bottom of the quiet waters and brings it to the surface, makes it shout above the others." (LISPECTOR, 1979, p. 77).

The metaphor of the hook has also been used by the author to fish for the reader - through her writing, she seeks to awaken quiet, dormant feelings in the reader, perhaps believing that facing them is a good way of not submitting to the suffering that many people cause us. The logic is similar to that of Daniel, who tells Cristina: "[...] Learn to enchant and disenchant. Look, I'm teaching you something precious: the magic opposite to 'open your eyes'. For a feeling to lose its perfume and stop intoxicating us, there's nothing better than exposing it to the sun." (LISPECTOR, 1979, p. 65). With regard to Clarice's writing, we understand that exposing the inner conflicts of human beings, their anguish, their helplessness, their finitude and their impossibility of representation are more effective ways of dealing with them than ignoring their existence.

The author exposes these feelings in countless ways, so the ways in which they arise in each individual are varied.

In the fourth story of *The Dehrio, the* reader can delve deeply into the complexity of the human mind, through the delusions of the protagonist, and also come into contact with pulsations. As an illustration of the death drive, we've chosen a passage from the narrative in which the narrator describes the protagonist's emotional state: "Where's the sun? Everything is dark, it's cold. There's a moment when he feels the darkness inside him, a vague desire to dilute himself, to disappear. You don't want to think, you can't think. Above all, you can't solve anything just yet - you put it off, you coward. He's still sick." (LISPECTOR, 1979, p. 93). We see there a desire to return to a nirvana-like, inanimate state, without excitements, at the same time as the character seeks the light which, in his case, seems to refer to the energy and vital force that sets him in motion, even leading him to write. The process of writing is thus described by the narrator:

> When he started, all his fibers crested, irritated, magnificent. And as long as he didn't cover the paper with nervous letters, as long as he didn't feel that they were his extension, he didn't stop, exhausting himself to the end... "The earth, the brave ones contracted with pain..." Yes, your head is already sore, heavy. But could she contain her light, to save herself?" (LISPECTOR, 1979, p. 94).

In this short story, we see creationist sublimation, according to Lacan's terminology, insofar as, faced with immanent destruction, the character renews himself, making the terrifying darkness and emptiness act as the driving force behind his artistic creation.

In the fifth story in the book, *The Escape,* we also identify this movement of creationist sublimation, through the creative daydreams of the protagonist character, against the imprisoning and meaningless reality in which she found herself. All she had to do was dream of a different reality and, through her dreams, find some comfort and a place for her desires. Because of this, the moment of dreaming, even though it is night, is described in the narrative as the moment of greatest illumination: "A great, pure light rises from the trees. He kept his eyes open for a while. Then she wiped her tears with o lengol, closed her eyes and got into bed. She feels the moonlight slowly covering her." (LISPECTOR, 1979, p. 104).

In most of the stories in the book, we notice the reiteration of antithetical words: light and dark, black and white, and we also associate them with the movements of life and death. It is common sense that light refers to life, coто confirm the expression "gave birth" to denote that the person has given birth to a child, that is, a new life; similarly, o black and darkness also refer to death. In this way, we can see that impulsive movements can be identified not only in the content of the text, but also in the "beyond" meanings that each word can contain and in the signifier, as the "sensory" part of the verbal sign. The repeated search for resources that point to meanings and make it possible to represent language is also indicative of the impossibility of representation, in other words, Clarice's writing recognizes emptiness and, precisely for this reason, tries to symbolize it, to produce something around it.

The creative movement from the void is recognized in the expression of language, in art, in the act of writing, but let's also remember that this movement is possible in the act of reading, since it is mainly from the voids in the text that the reader is summoned to create and fill in the gaps with their fantasies and desires. This is what we see in the sixth story in the book, *Two More Drunkards, when* the narrative ends abruptly and the reader is invited to construct meanings for its ending.

In the short story *Two more drunks,* the reader's quest to understand how the narrative ends is similar to the protagonist's quest to understand death and the finitude inherent in human life. The protagonist's dialogue with the stranger he meets in the bar is also an attempt at a dialogue with the reader; it's an invitation to reflect on this human question with him. Let's read it:

> [...] Don't you suffer, friend? I... I can't stand it. It hurts me here, in the center of my heart. To have to die one day and, thousands of centuries later, undifferentiated in humus, with no eyes for the rest of eternity, I, ME, with no eyes for the rest of eternity... and the moon indifferent and triumphant, pale hands outstretched over new men, new things, other beings. And me Dead!" I breathed deeply. - Think, my friend. Right now she's over the cemetery too. The cemetery, where all those who have been and never will be sleep. There, where the slightest whisper sends a shiver of terror through the living and where the tranquillity of the stars muzzles our screams and stares into our eyes. There, where there are no tears or thoughts to express the profound misery of ending (LISPECTOR, 1979, p. 113).

The condition of mortality is recurrently exposed in the short stories and also throughout Clarice's work. In one of her novels, *The Passion According to G.H.,* the author writes: "I'll tell you a secret: life is mortal." (LISPECTOR, 1998b, p. 77). And this secret, kept absolutely secret from ourselves, makes sense in the face of the strangeness and anguish it provokes when reading a text that refers to such a condition.

The strangeness of the reader in the act of reading and the effect of art on its observer are important aspects in examining the process of subjectivation and the construction of identities. As we have already said, the cooperative and dialectical interaction between reader and literary text, this bond created coто potential interpretations and effects, is an intimate encounter that leads to transformation for both reader and text.

As an illustration of this process, we turn to the last story, *Beauty and the Beast or The Wound That's Too Big,* in which the protagonist Carla de Souza e Santos compares the revelation she gained in her encounter with the beggar to a revelation she had also gained through art. Let's see: "She was as frightened as she had been when she saw Mona Lisa's smile, there, holding her hand in the Louvre. Just as she had been frightened by the man in the wound or the wound in the man." (LISPECTOR, 1979, p. 141). She also remembers her childhood, when she took singing lessons and how listening to classical music also took her out of the "automatic sleep in which she lived". The protagonist reflects: "This story of looking for art in order to understand had only happened to her once - then she had sunk into a forgetfulness that only now, at the age of thirty-five, through the wound, did she have to either sing very badly or sing very well - she was bewildered." (LISPECTOR, 1979, p. 146). In this way, the story draws attention to the possibility of revelation by other means, not only through the encounter with otherness, but also through the impact and revelation of reality through art.

We believe that the short story *Beauty and the Beast or The Wound Too Big* closes the book *Beauty and the Beast* by condensing the most important and recurring aspects in the plots of the other short stories in the book, and that the encounter with otherness is an important process in the formation of identity; the presence of an event that marks the life of a character so that they can no longer be the same; the tireless search by Clarice's characters for a more authentic life; literature as a possible revelation of the real, enabling the ordering of psychic chaos and, consequently, enabling the process of subjectivation.

FINAL CONSIDERATIONS

But you have to be clever
And you need to be funny
And I need you always
Who bears this mark on their skin
I have a strange habit
To have faith in life (MILTONNASCIMENTO,1978)

Up to this point, we have traveled tortuous, often obscure paths, full of deconstructions, starting with the deconstruction of the idea of the Cartesian cogito, restricted to the registers of the field of consciousness and reason, considering the self сото an original and totalizing instance of the psyche. From the deconstruction of this idea and the recognition of an ego that needs to be developed, it was necessary to consider the need for an other and, consequently, the recognition of otherness is fundamental to the subject in their process of subjectivation. This other gains importance by playing an organizing role in the chaos of impulses in which the subject finds himself, which was made possible by the deconstruction of a neutral self, i.e. the discovery of a self invested with sexuality and full of impulses. In this way, the idea of an organized subject, ordered by vital instincts, falls apart when Freud discovers the existence of a drive without representation, which produces rupture and dispersion.

These deconstructions have affected literature in a big way, as we have debunked the idea that the text contains only one truth; in fact, the literary text is a space that allows for countless interpretations and, even so, is incapable of conveying all that reality entails. We've seen that literature recognizes the limits of representation and language, as well as the lack and emptiness that make up the subject, but it doesn't paralyze itself in the face of this; on the contrary, it makes these "deconstructions" and impossibilities its force for movement and creation. Therein lies Clarice's writing, which oscillates between deadly and vital movements, bringing up the themes of anguish and helplessness, without losing sight of the search for symbolization, creation and encounter. As we see in the trajectory of his characters, who, faced with the existential anguish resulting from not knowing themselves, often seek new guidelines and possible happiness through writing, which consequently pushes Lambern o the reader to seek new paths and alternatives after coming into contact with the "disorientation" of these readings.

Emilia Amaral (2005), referring to Clarice Lispector's novel *Paixao segundo G. H.,* sums up the reader's feeling towards Clarice's texts in the same way that we also identify with after reading the short stories in *Beauty and the Beast.* She says:

> To come into contact with Clarice's text, to be touched by it, would require, according to these words (I'm thinking of the combination of note and epigraph), "readers with an already formed soul", in other words, readers prepared for a journey towards disorganization, absorption, dissolution and death, which is, for this very reason, "rejuvenating". (AMARAL, 2005, p. 25).

In fact, we went through deconstructions, disagreements, and came into contact with the anguish of helplessness and human finitude. However, we were enlivened by the contact with new spaces, the unconscious, affections, desire and fantasies, the intimacy of the encounter with the other, the alternative of many identities instead of just one, the viability of producing many truths instead of just one; in short, we were enlivened by the possibility of creation in the face of imminent destruction. Revived by hope, by a strange faith in life...

[0]Recognizing this tragic aspect of life, the poet Ferreira Gullar addresses the issue of individual creation in the face of the helplessness of existence and writes a chronicle published in the newspaper *Folha de S.Paulo.* dated January 1, 2006, entitled *Um bicho que se inventa.* in which he says:

> Human society was invented by our ancestors. Anyone born today finds it already invented, materially and spiritually, with the equipment, values and principles that make it up and define it. It is within this complex and contradictory cultural reality that they will invent themselves as a unique and unmistakable individual. Because each of us wants to be like that; unique and unmistakable. To **live is therefore to invent oneself: to invent one's life, one's function in the world, one's presence** (GULLAR, 2006, *online,* emphasis added).

We believe that staging the possibility of "inventing" ourselves every day and every moment is the greatest contribution that art can make to our work in the search to understand the process of constructing identity in relation to the other, as well as the search by each of us to be unique and unmistakable. It's a constant, necessary search, which makes it possible to keep moving, as Clarice describes in her book *Agua Viva.* "What I'm writing to you is an 'it'. It won't stop: it goes on." (LISPECTOR, 1980. p. 87).

In this sense, our work does not end here, despite the period. It continues.

REFERENCES

AMARAL, Emilia. O **leitor segundo G. H.:** uma analise do romance *A paixao segundo G.H. de* Clarice Lispector. Cotia: Atelie Editorial, 2005.

AREAS, Vilma. **Clarice Lispector at your fingertips.** Sao Paulo: Companhia das Letras, 2005.

BELLEMIN-NOEL, Jean. **Psychoanalysis and Literature.** Translated by Alvaro Lorenci and Sandra Nitrini. São Paulo: Ed. Cultrix, 1983.

BIRMAN, Joel. Bodies and forms of subjectivation in psychoanalysis. In: GENERAL STATES OF PSYCHOANALYSIS: WORLD MEETING, 2, 2003a. Rio de Janeiro. **Proceedings...** 1-36 p.
Available at: <http://egp.dreamhosters.com/encontros/mundial rj/download/3 Birman 38020903 port.pdfAccessed: Nov. 10, 2013.

BIRMAN, Joel. **Freud and philosophy.** Rio de Janeiro: Jorge Zahar. Ed, 2003b.

BORELLI, Olga. **Clarice Lispector: sketch for a possible portrait.** Rio de Janeiro: Nova Fronteira. 1981.

CAMPOS, Paulo Mendes. **Conversations with Clarice.** Close to Clarice. Rio de Janeiro: Casa de Cultura Laura Alvim, 1987. (Catalogue).

CANDIDO, Antonio. **No comedo era de fato o verbo.** In: NUNES, B. (Coord.) A paixao Segundo G.H: edigao critica. Madrid; Paris; Mexico; Buenos Aires; Sao Paulo; Rio de Janeiro; Lima: ALLCA XX, 1996. (Coleccion Archives: 2 ed.; 13)

CANDIDO, Antonio. **Vanos escritos.** Sao Paulo: Duas Cidades; Rio de Janeiro: Ouro sobre Azul, 2004. p.169-191.

CUNHA, Eduardo Leal. A psychoanalytic interrogation of identities. **Caderno CRH,** Salvador, n. 33, p. 209-228, Jul./Dec. 2000.

CUNHA, Eduardo Leal. The **singular and plural individual:** a psychoanalytic critique of identities. 2005. 228f. Thesis (Doctorate in Mental Health) - State University of Rio de Janeiro, Institute of Social Medicine, Rio de Janeiro, 2005.

ECO, Umberto. **Open Work.** Sao Paulo: Perspective 2003.

FERREIRA, Aurelio Buarque de Holanda. **Dicionario da Lingua Portuguesa.** Rio de Janeiro: Positive, 2010.

FREITAS, Jane Pinheiro. **Before the Beginning Was the Word:** a reading of Clarice Lispector's Beauty and the Beast. 2002. 120 f. Dissertation (Master's in Literature) - University of Sao Paulo, Sao Paulo, 2002.

FREUD, Sigmund. Project for a scientific psychology. In: FREUD, Sigmund. **Pre-psychoanalytic publications and unpublished sketches.** Rio de Janeiro: Imago, 1996a. p. 333-443 (Brazilian standard edition of the complete psychological works of Sigmund Freud: volume 1).

FREUD, Sigmund. Forms on the two principles of mental functioning. In: FREUD, Sigmund. O **Schereber case, Articles on technique and other works.** Rio de Janeiro: Imago, 1996b. p. 233-244. (Brazilian Standard Edition of the Complete Psychological Works of Sigmund Freud: Volume 7).

FREUD, Sigmund. Fragments of the analysis of a case of hysteria. In: FREUD, Sigmund. **A Case of Hysteria, Three Essays on Sexuality and other works.** Rio de Janeiro: Imago, 1996b. p. 15-116 (Brazilian Standard Edition of the Complete Psychological Works of Sigmund Freud: Volume 7).

FREUD, Sigmund. Three essays on the theory of sexuality. In: FREUD, Sigmund. **A case of hysteria, three essays on sexuality and other works.** Rio de Janeiro: Imago, 1996b. 119-151p. (Brazilian Standard Edition of the Complete Psychological Works of Sigmund Freud: Volume 7)

FREUD, Sigmund. Creative writers and reverie. In: FREUD, Sigmund. **Jensen's Gradiva and other works.** Rio de Janeiro: Imago, 1996c. p. 133-143. (Brazilian Standard Edition of the Complete Psychological Works of Sigmund Freud: Volume 9).

FREUD, Sigmund. Leonardo da Vinci and a memory of his childhood. In: FREUD, Sigmund. **Five Lessons in Psychoanalysis, Leonardo da Vinci and other works.** Rio de Janeiro: Imago, 1996d. p. 67-141. (Brazilian Standard Edition of the Complete Psychological Works of Sigmund Freud: Volume 11).

FREUD, Sigmund. **The history of the psychoanalytic movement, articles on metapsychology and other works.** Rio de Janeiro: Imago, 1996e. (Standard Brazilian edition of the complete psychological works of Sigmund Freud: volume 14).

FREUD, Sigmund. The instincts and their vicissitudes. In: FREUD, Sigmund. **The history of the psychoanalytic movement, articles on metapsychology and other works.** Rio de Janeiro: Imago, 1996e. p. 117-144. (Brazilian Standard Edition of the Complete Psychological Works of Sigmund Freud: Volume 14).

FREUD, Sigmund. On narcissism: an introduction. In: FREUD, Sigmund. **The history of the psychoanalytic movement, articles on metapsychology and other works.** Rio de Janeiro: Imago, 1996e. p. 77-108. (Brazilian Standard Edition of the Complete Psychological Works of Sigmund Freud: Volume 14).

FREUD, Sigmund. O stranger. In: FREUD, Sigmund. **An infantile neurosis and other works.** Rio de Janeiro: Imago, 1996f. p. 237-273 (Brazilian Standard Edition of the Complete Psychological Works of Sigmund Freud: Volume 17)

FREUD, Sigmund. A difficulty on the road to psychoanalysis. In: FREUD, Sigmund. **An infantile neurosis and other works.** Rio de Janeiro: Imago, 1996f. p. 145-167. (Brazilian Standard Edition of the Complete Psychological Works of Sigmund Freud: Volume 17).

FREUD, Sigmund. The pleasure principle. In: FREUD, Sigmund. **Beyond the pleasure principle, Group Psychology and other works.** Rio de Janeiro: Imago, 1996g. p. 13-75. (Brazilian Standard Edition of the Complete Psychological Works of Sigmund Freud: Volume 18).

FREUD, Sigmund. O malaise in civilization. In: FREUD, Sigmund. O **future of an Illusion, O malaise in civilization and other works.** Rio de Janeiro: Imago, 1996h. p. 67148. (Brazilian Standard Edition of the Complete Psychological Works of Sigmund Freud: Volume 21).

GOTLIB, Nadia Batella. **Clarice:** a life that can be told. 6. ed. Sao Paulo: Editora da Universidade de Sao Paulo, 2009.

GOULART, Audemaro Taranto. **Topics in Portuguese Literature.** Belo Horizonte: Postgraduate Program in Letters, PUC Minas, 2012. (Handout).

GREEN, Andre. O **disconnection:** psychoanalysis, anthropology and literature. Translated by Irene Cubric. Rio de Janeiro: Imago, 1994.

HOFFMANN, E.T.A. O **man of the sand.** In: Fantastic tales. Rio de Janeiro: Imago, 1993. p.113-147.

LACAN, Jacques. O **Seminar, Book 7, The Ethics of Psychoanalysis.** Rio de Janeiro: Jorge Zahar Editor, 1988.

LACAN, Jacques. The signification of the phallus. In: LACAN, Jacques. **Writings.** Rio de Janeiro: Jorge Zahar, 1998.

LISPECTOR, Clarice. **Near the Wild Heart.** Rio de Janeiro, ANoite, 1943.

LISPECTOR, Clarice. **The Foreign Legion.** Rio de Janeiro: Editora do Autor, 1964.

LISPECTOR, Clarice. **Agua Viva.** Rio de Janeiro: Artenova, 1973.

LISPECTOR, Clarice. **A breath of life:** pulsagoes. Rio de Janeiro: Nova Fronteira, 1978.

LISPECTOR, Clarice. **Beauty and the Beast.** Rio de Janeiro: Nova Fronteira, 1979.

LISPECTOR, Clarice. **Agua Viva.** 4. ed. Rio de Janeiro: Nova Fronteira, 1980.

LISPECTOR, Clarice. **La?os de familia:** contos. Rio de Janeiro: Francisco Alves, 1994.

LISPECTOR, Clarice. **The hour of the star.** Rio de Janeiro: Rocco, 1998a.

LISPECTOR, Clarice. **A paixao segundo G. H.:** romance. Rio de Janeiro: Rocco; 1998b.

LISPECTOR, Clarice. **The discovery of the world.** Rio de Janeiro: Rocco. 1999a.

LISPECTOR, Clarice. **A Breath of Life (Pulsa^oes).** Rio de Janeiro: Rocco, 1999b.

MANGUEL, Alberto. **A history of reading.** Translated by Pedro Maia Soares. São Paulo: Companhiadas Letras, 1997.

MORAES, Ddbora Ferreira Leite. **Psychoanalytic essay for a metapsychology of the literary reader:** a reading of *Agua Viva* by Clarice Lispector. 2011.133 f. Dissertation (Master's in Psychology) - University of Sao Paulo, 2011, Sao Paulo.

MOREIRA, Jaqueline de Oliveira. Revisiting Freud's concept of the self: from identity to alterity. **Estudos e Pesquisa em Psicologia,** Rio de Janeiro, ano 9, n. 1, p. 233-247, jan./jul. 2009. Available at: <http://www.revispsi.ueri.br/v9nl/artigos/pdf7v9nlal8.pdf.>. Accessed: Dec. 10,

2013.

NUNES, Benedito. O **drama da linguagem** - uma leitura de Clarice Lispector. Atica, 1989.

OGDEN, Thomas. **The subjects of psychoanalysis.** Translated by Claudia Berlinet. Sao Paulo: Casa do Psicologo, 1996.

PELLEGRINO, Helio. Oedipus and passion. In: PELLEGRINO, helio et al. **Os sentidos da paixao.** São Paulo: Companhia das Letras, 1987. p. 307-327.

PONTIERI, Regina. Visions of otherness: Clarice Lispector and Maurice Merleau-Ponty. **Revista USP,** Sao Paulo, n. 44, p. 330-334, Dec./Feb. 1999.

ROCHA, Zeferino. **The destinies of anguish in Freudian psychoanalysis.** Sao Paulo: Escuta. 2000.

ROSEMBAUM, Youdith. **The metamorphoses of evil** (A reading of Clarice Lispector). 1997. 293 f. Thesis (Doctorate in Philosophy, Letters and Human Sciences) - University of Sao Paulo, Sao Paulo, 1997.

ROSENBAUM, Yudith. **Metamorphoses of evil:** a reading of Clarice Lispector. Sao Paulo: Editora da Universidade de Sao Paulo: Fapesp, 1999.

ROUDINESCO, Elisabeth; PLON, Michel. **Dictionary of psychoanalysis.** Rio de Janeiro: J. Zahar, 1998.

SAMPAIO, Camila Pedral. The impact of literature on psychoanalytic interpretation. In: BARTUCCI, Giovanna (Org.). **Psychoanalysis, art and aesthetics of subjectivity.** Rio de Janeiro: Imago Ed., 2002. p. 153-175.

SAMPAIO, Camila Pedral. Conjugates between psychoanalysis and literature. In: BARONE, Leda Maria (Coord.). **psychoanalysis and the extensive clinic:** III psychoanalytic meeting of field theory in writing. Sao Paulo: Casa do Psicologo, 2005.

SANT'ANNA, Affonso Romano de. **Structural analysis of Brazilian novels.** 7. ed. Sao Paulo, Atica, 1990.

TEIXEIRA, Leonia Cavalcante. O lugar da literatura na constituigao da clinica psicanalitica em Freud. **Psyche,** Sao Paulo, v. 9, n. 16, dec. 2005. Available at: <http://pepsic.bvsalud. org/scielo.php?script=sci_arttext&pid=S1415-11382005000200008&lng=en&nrm=iso>. Accessed on: 26 Dec. 2013.

VALLE, Ana Maria Lima do. **Clarice Lispector's Writing in the Transmission of the Real.** 2006. 117f. Dissertation (Master's in Psychology) - Institute of Psychology, Rio de Janeiro State University, Rio de Janeiro, 2006.

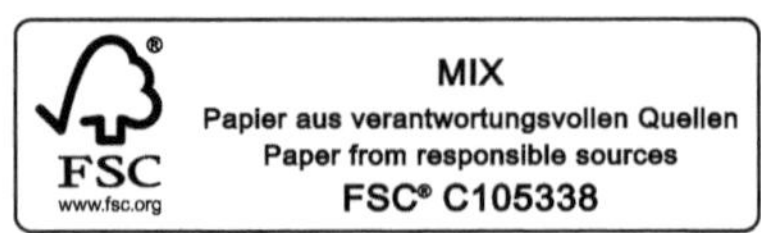

Printed by Books on Demand GmbH, Norderstedt / Germany